THE STUDENT DOCTOR NETWORK®

Dental School Admissions Guide

GURPREET S. KHURANA, DMD

The Student Doctor Network®
www.studentdoctor.net

SDN ACADEMIC PRESS

The Student Doctor Network Dental School Admissions Guide
by Gurpreet S. Khurana, DMD

Copyright © 2010 by Gurpreet S. Khurana, DMD

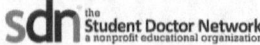

www.studentdoctor.net

Published and distributed by
SDN ACADEMIC PRESS

All rights reserved. No part of this book may be used or reproduced in any manner whatsoever without written permission except for brief quotations embodied in critical articles and reviews.

The SDN Logo and "The Student Doctor Network" are registered trademarks of the Coastal Research Group. The Student Doctor Network® and SDN Academic Press are operated as a public service by the Coastal Research Group, a 501(c)3 charitable organization.

Printed in the United States of America

For information write:
SDN ACADEMIC PRESS
16835 Algonquin Street #308
Huntington Beach, CA 92649

ISBN 13: 978-0-9833962-0-8

ACKNOWLEDGMENTS

This book is dedicated to my parents, Rani and Gurpal.

Table of Contents

ACKNOWLEDGMENTS i
PREFACE 1
HOW TO USE THIS GUIDE 3
WHY DENTAL SCHOOL? 4
WHO GOES TO DENTAL SCHOOL? 7
THE GAME PLAN 8
THE PRE-DENTAL YEARS: HIGH SCHOOL AND COLLEGE. 9
       COLLEGE YEARS 11
THE DENTAL ADMISSION TEST 16
THE DENTAL APPLICATION 43
THE DENTAL ESSAY: YOUR SELF PORTRAIT 50
       SAMPLE ADMISSION ESSAYS 52
       THE NON-TRADITIONAL APPLICANT 61
       POST-BACCALAUREATE PROGRAMS: 63
CANADIAN DENTAL APPLICANTS 70
THE INTERVIEW 74
       COMMON INTERVIEW QUESTIONS 75
110 QUESTIONS ABOUT DENTAL SCHOOL 85
YOU GOT IN – NOW WHAT?? 121
DENTAL TERMINOLOGY 123
LIST OF DENTAL SCHOOLS IN THE UNITED STATES 136
FINANCING YOUR DENTAL EDUCATION 177
FOR INTERNATIONAL DENTAL CANDIDATES 186
DENTAL SCHOOLS WITH
       ADVANCED STANDING PROGRAMS 187
DENTAL ETHICS 198
BIBLIOGRAPHY 207

INTERNET RESOURCES 207
SOME USEFUL LINKS FOR PRE-DENTAL STUDENTS 208
INDEX 209

PREFACE

As a pre-dental student, I came across a huge problem finding information about dental school. While there were many sources available, I quickly realized, to my dismay, that there was not one single resource that explained how to thoroughly prepare for the dental school application process. Yes, there were resources written by Ph.D's that were not up-to-date, or others that explained a different viewpoint than that of a traditional applicant.

When I began visiting dental programs and asked school advisors for answers to my questions, I encountered another problem: most of them had no clue about the admissions process. They would often compare the dental school application process to medical school, and would give information that was similar, but not pertinent to me. They had ample knowledge about medical admissions, but it was evident that there was a huge disparity.

Dentists are in high demand. The opportunities are endless and slowly, people are realizing the benefits of pursuing a career in dentistry. I believe that competition will be at an all time high. Competition for seats in dental admissions will soon meet, if not exceed, medical school. Some schools are already beginning to see higher competition for their entering dental school class, than their medical school according to ADEA released statistics. These trends will become increasingly apparent in the near future.

Over the next decade about half of the currently 150,000 working dentists are projected to retire, leaving a huge gap to be filled. As the population grows, and the baby boomer population doubles, the need for oral health care professionals will be at an all time high. Some states are experiencing a huge decline in dentists, with some areas experiencing retirement of 10 dentists for every one new dentist entering the workforce.

For the past six years, I have compiled, discussed, and researched all aspects of the pre-dental lifestyle and want to present to fellow pre-dental students, advanced-standing students, and current dental students a complete guide for their reference. I believe students can depend on this publication as their main resource.

I will explain all aspects from an applicant's standpoint, since I recently completed this process, graduated dental school, passed the boards, and am now a practicing dentist. The process of applying to dental school is rigorous and demanding. Therefore, I wish to utilize and share the resources that I have found most helpful to provide new students with the information they need.

I wish you complete success in your dental endeavors.

G.S. Khurana, DMD

HOW TO USE THIS GUIDE

This guide is written with all types of applicants in mind. From those who have known that they wanted to be in the dental profession from childhood, to adults who want to change their career. The simple approach of this guide is to give everyone a fair understanding of what it takes to be a dentist. This guide will share the basics which many people already know, and will also bring forth ideas and information that others may have never heard of. The best way to utilize this guide is to skim each chapter or section. Keep it handy and skim through it during a commercial break or on the bus. Each time, you may find something useful about the application process.

Once you begin the application process it is advisable for you to read and understand all parts of the guide, as there are worksheets that will help you brainstorm your ideas about give you tips on successfully tackling the application process.

Do not be afraid to highlight, scribble notes, and make this guide your personal dental application journal. Once you finish dental school and are a practicing dentist, you may just pick it up after all the hurdles and reflect on where you started and where you ended up. Also, if you have to re-apply, this guide will serve as a way to look back on your previous application, helping you submit a much stronger application the year after.

- Skim through the guide during any free time you have
- Prior to beginning the application cycle, read the guide thoroughly
- Highlight and make notes
- Complete all worksheets in the guide

WHY DENTAL SCHOOL?

Dentistry is one of the hottest professions in the United States and this can be proven by comparing the lifestyles of dentists and other health care professionals. According to the ADA, the average general dentist's net income from primary private practice was $185,000 in 2004. The average specialist's net income was $315,000. You might think dentists put in a lot of hours with salaries like that. On the contrary, according to the American Dental Association the average work week of a dentist is 35–37 hours a week! That is almost half of a typical physician's work week, which is often 60 to 80 hours a week. Over 90% of dental professionals own their own practice and therefore have autonomy and less stress.

However, just like everything that is worth having in life, one must be willing to sacrifice for it. Becoming a dentist requires passion, belief, and a plan of action. You must be willing to give long hours and be persistent. Dentistry, unlike other professions, requires a lot out of the individual who wants to embark on this journey leading to dental school and beyond. A dentist needs to be an entrepreneur, good with his/her hands, artistic, a leader, and an organized and compassionate individual. To become a successful dentist, these qualities are a must have.

Dentistry has changed a lot in the past few decades. The main goal of dentistry has taken more of a preventative and cosmetic aspect to it, whereas several decades ago, people would go to a dentist only when they experience discomfort or extreme pain. Today, the average person goes to a dentist at least twice a year for a routine checkup. Extracting a tooth is the last resort. The goal is to save one's permanent dentition so it can last a lifetime. In third-world countries it is not uncommon to see people having all their teeth extracted before the age of 50; however, in the United States there is a new trend to save the permanent dentition. Elderly citizens go through various lengths to avoid wearing dentures. Now, technologies such as implants, crowns, root canal therapies, and orthodontics have revolutionized the tooth saving power of dentists.

As the baby boomer generation begins to retire and expand, dentists will have a plethora of patients on their hands who, when they were young, neglected their dental care, but during retirement want to regain that youthful smile they once took for granted. Also, this baby boomer generation will have more disposable income saved up from decades of working. With the population and oral health awareness growing exponentially and many dentists retiring, there will be more work than all the dentists can handle.

Dentistry is not only mentally challenging but also physically demanding. Working in such a small area such as the mouth can be a challenge, especially with a powerful drill buzzing around 100,000 RPM. It is a profession of precision. When teeth preparations are a few millimeters, it takes a controlled individual to operate new technologies such as lasers and drills. Do not let this scare you. Oral health professionals help people every day. From preventing cavities, to taking care of pain, they do it all. As a dentist you will understand the importance of prevention, as well as taking care of emergency situations.

Dentists also save lives. They diagnose oral cancer and jaw pathology during regular exams. A competent dentist can save someone's life if a small oral lesion is detected early. Every year tens of thousands of people are diagnosed with oral cancer, many of them are detected by dentists who were thorough and found the lesion early.

ଛ ଓ

One of the newest and most fascinating trends in dentistry is cosmetics. Dentists can transform patients' smiles through various new technologies including Invisalign® with clear braces, CEREC® for immediate milling of crowns and veneers, and laser bleaching technologies such as ZOOM!®. Not only do these technologies give amazing results, but they are also very fast acting. Just a few years ago, crowns would take two to four weeks and several appointments to fit; now patients can come in and in as little as an hour, they can leave with a permanent crown. Braces have become invisible. Who knew? People with stained, yellow teeth can brighten their smile in one hour. All of these technologies have made dentistry one of the most popular career fields right now.

Right now you may be trying to finish your requirements or have recently completed them, and are wondering which profession to choose. The next section will discuss how to take advantage of the pre-dental years and how you can successfully get into dental school.

ഈ ൚

WHO GOES TO DENTAL SCHOOL?

Now that you have picked up this book, you may ask yourself: So who goes to dental school? Are all applicants like me?

Dentistry is a profession that combines various realms which every applicant needs to be aware of prior to applying. After reflecting on what dentistry is, you may have realized that it's not only about dealing with people's oral health, it's much more. Dentistry is a combination of healthcare, art, and business. To be a successful dentist, you must understand that the combination of art and science is crucial in treating patients. Working with your hands and excellent dexterity is essential. Many dentists are perfectionists because in the mouth a few millimeters can make a huge difference.

Most dentists own their own practice so they must not only understand how to treat patients, but how to manage an office and its staff. In addition, knowing basic accounting and marketing skills will help you in this profession. However, the most essential ingredients that a dentist must possess are passion and empathy. Anyone who chooses dentistry as a profession must realize that without passion for the field, or empathy or patients, failure is likely to occur.

In summary, who goes into the field of dentistry?

One that loves to work with his/her hands, as well as one that loves the combination of art, science, and business while treating patients in an empathetic manner.

THE GAME PLAN

Pre-Dental Years
- Maintain good grades in all of your classes. Earn at least a 3.5 GPA.
- Diversify your class experience. Take a variety of classes in different subjects of interest.
- Keep an eye on the prerequisite classes for dental school.
- Get experience in the dental field. Find a mentor to guide you and answer your questions about dentistry so you know what you are getting yourself into.

The Application Cycle
- Have three good recommendations ready to go prior to the application cycle.
- Write your essay and have it proofread by colleagues and professors.
- Take your DAT early.
- Apply early.

Interviews
- Practice all interview questions with friends
- Be confident and maintain a sharp appearance.

Post-acceptance
- Celebrate!
- Review financial aid information.
- Enjoy your summer prior to matriculation.

ಸಿ ಅ

THE PRE-DENTAL YEARS: HIGH SCHOOL AND COLLEGE.

So you've decided to consider a career in dentistry. It's a noble and intensely rewarding profession that involves more than just filling and cleaning teeth. By now you've figured out you have an interest, and want to explore the profession in depth. Perhaps you are wondering where it may lead, and how you can get there. For those who are still in high school, you have started the journey into dentistry early, and beginning early can be one of the best ways to get started. If you have decided that dentistry is for you, then you can begin mapping out a plan of action as to how you can get into a proper college – one that can prepare you for dental school.

In order to truly get an idea of what the practice of dental medicine is all about, the best piece of advice any dental student, professor, or advisor can give you is to start shadowing a dentist. Nothing can replace firsthand experience. If you do not know a dentist personally, don't hesitate to find one in your area and call them. Many of the dentists who are in practice are extremely approachable and helpful, and are keen to show you their world. First, introduce yourself, and then tell them you're considering a career in dentistry and want exposure. You just want to sit and watch the dentist perform procedures, but if you are lucky, (or if you have more experience) the dentist may want you to help. This can mean many things: they may want you to sterilize or organize instruments, or even help you sort charts. All of these things are important to learn since a dentist not only works on patients but understand the business of dentistry. Once you have mastered these, you may even get to assist the dentist. While assisting, you will gain a lot of insight on what dentistry is about.

While you're still in high school and immersing yourself in the world of dentistry, you should continue to pursue a curriculum that will give you a solid foundation in science. This will be extremely beneficial to you when you enter college, and will help you reinforce necessary materials that you will encounter in dental school. Remember, the more you see the information, the easier it is to remember it. If you're doing well in school, are finding that shadowing a dentist is intriguing and rewarding, and are ready to commit yourself to the profession, then there are a couple of options for you. The most traditional approach to getting into dental school is to graduate from high school, attend college, obtain a Bachelor's degree, and then go to dental school. This route generally takes between seven and eight years for the average student. The other approach is to apply straight from high school to universities that have accelerated programs. Many medical schools in the U.S. have six and seven year medical programs that combine an undergraduate degree with a medical degree, and there are some universities that offer this approach to dental school.

If you aren't sure what career path to follow, or even if you find dentistry fascinating, attending college for four years can put a lot of things into perspective, give you a chance to learn about other disciplines, and see if dentistry is truly right for you. For those of you who still can't see anything other than working as a dentist, applying to the accelerated programs is for you!

సౌ ౧ౠ

COLLEGE YEARS

While you're attending college, the best thing you can do is to continue learning about dentistry. Many schools have a dental clinic, a dental ER, or a private practice clinic near the school. Take the first step and volunteer. The more time you spend, the more you will learn. Another key point is that although you may have a solid interest, deep fascination, and a striking desire to pursue dentistry, you must find other things to do outside the realm of dental medicine. Find other interests, hobbies, and activities that will make your college experience enriching. Involving yourself in different types of organizations and clubs will give you a well-rounded experience. Often people forget that dentistry is a subspecialty of medicine. As you learn more about medicine, you will educate yourself and will in turn, become more certain that dentistry is the profession you want to pursue. To become a dentist, you must be empathetic. If this is not something that comes natural to you, it can be learned by participating in food drives, working at homeless shelters, or volunteering in nursing homes. At the end, you are not just taking care of a tooth, but the whole person. So the more you understand and work with people, the better of a dentist you will become. Once you learn how to connect with people and understand them, you will understand that dentistry encompasses a lot more than drilling on teeth.

Picking a major can be another pitfall for college students. Many people will tell you that the majority of students entering dental school (any health profession school, for that matter) majored in biology. But that doesn't mean that it's vital, critical, or remotely essential to major in biology. There are prerequisites are required to enter dental school regardless of your major, so this is your opportunity to study other fields of interest you might have. For example, if you have a keen interest in music or languages, you may consider majoring in music or a language. This will surely introduce you to a vast amount of people who may not be just pre-healthcare students. Also, majoring in something you are interested in will give you an advantage, in that your grades may be higher and admissions committees in dental schools will be curious about your choice of major. Several of my classmates were classics majors, business majors, and even theater majors. No dental school will reject you because you majored in something that interested you. Variety is good, and if you study something you have a genuine interest in, you are bound to excel. However, there are courses that are required in order to be admitted to dental school and ones that will give you the foundation for the Dental Admission Test. It is mandatory that these classes be completed. Some of these include: General Chemistry, Organic Chemistry, Biology, Physics, Biochemistry, Calculus, and English. These are just the general requirements, but each school has a list of specific requirements and suggested courses. While it may appear to be a lot of classes (and it is!) it is totally manageable if you are organized. The reason many people decide to major in Biology or any other science is because many of the classes that are required for dental school admission are required for the major, which therefore allows for a more efficient use of time and resources. In addition, these classes are also where the foundation will be laid for the DAT. (The DAT is also known as the Dental Admission Test which is a requirement prior to matriculating to any U.S. dental school.)

For many students thinking about taking the DAT, they worry that their weaknesses in certain classes will prevent them from doing well on the DAT. This could not be further from the truth! Students may also worry about trying to keep up with class competition. Although most of the students who are pre-dental are relatively calm and easy going, the competition is always increasing. Most students are not malicious by nature, but they are competitive, and nobody wants to be at a disadvantage. Preparing for the DAT by yourself will not be detrimental to your performance, as long as you keep up with the material and study earnestly. Another issue that comes up is the debate of which review materials are better. Whether you buy the Kaplan or Princeton

Review material (or any other review material on the market today), the most important part to remember is that you must recall the information, mechanisms, and you need the ability to finish the test within the allotted time limit. Many students sign up for expensive review courses, and do well. But many dental students in dental school will tell you that these courses are not absolutely necessary (although, they may provide you with peace of mind).

The following is a basic format of what your first years of college should look like:

Year One
   English class (one to two semesters)
   Math class (one to two semesters)
   Biology or Chemistry (two semesters)

Year Two
   Chemistry or Biology (two semesters)
   Physics (two semesters)
   Select a major
   Start observing dentists

Year Three
   Organic Chemistry (two semesters)
   Study for the DAT (six to eight weeks)
   Obtain three solid recommendation letters
   Apply to dental school in the summer
   Continue to get dental experience

Year Four
   Go to interviews
   Finish your degree(s)
   Graduate

The schedule above is generic, and encompasses the basic prerequisites. Once you select your major you will fill the major requirements around these classes. You may even want to switch the core classes (Biology, Chemistry, or Physics) around as different schools may want you to take one core sequence first. For example, you may need to take first year of general chemistry prior to taking biology. Almost all schools require you to take General Chemistry before Organic Chemistry. You can also take physics your fourth year, but it is wise to take it prior to applying, so dental schools know that you are done with all your requirements. Once accepted, dental schools will want your final transcript and proof of diploma, showing that you completed all required courses successfully. If you have completed everything prior to applying, it will show the dental admissions committee that you have achieved basic competence in getting ready for the rigors of dental school.

Once you are at the stage of organizing your school schedule, you may want to sit down with an academic advisor. But before you do this, make sure you understand the basic requirements of dental school. Many academic advisors may think dental school admission is similar to medical school. This may be partially true, but you should ask if they understand the application process and have helped other pre-dental students gain admission. You and the advisor will then sit down and structure your course schedule so it is not overwhelming and contradictory.

The next step is to complete a standardized test called the Dental Admissions Test. This is a good way to show the dental school admissions committee that you have the basic understanding of the core classes. You may wonder why the DAT is necessary when you have earned all A's and B's in your classes. Well, a standardized test is to put all applicants on a level playing field. It is hard to evaluate thousands of dental applicants based on grades alone. Student A may have done all his or her prerequisites at community college and earned all A's, while student B attended an Ivy League school and received all B's and C's. The Dental Admission Test equalizes the candidates. Regardless, getting A's is ideal, but if you went to a competitive undergraduate institution and had a hard time getting all A's, then you have a chance to show the admissions committee that you are a capable dental student by passing the DAT. Regardless, your grade point average is very important. It is by far the most important requirement for successful dental school admission and should not be taken lightly. You should aim to earn at least a 3.5 average GPA and a 3.3 in sciences alone. Remember, the higher GPA you have, the more selection you will have for dental school.

ಸಾ ಡ

THE DENTAL ADMISSION TEST

The DAT is the Dental Admissions Test. It is a standardized test that all students who are pursuing admission to dental school must take. You may wonder what's on the DAT. Remember that list of general required classes? Well, many of the subjects that were required for dental admission show up on the DAT. However, not all of the information you studied will be on the DAT. Below is a simple synopsis of the topics that will be found on the DAT, as well as examples of some questions that you'll see in each section:

Perceptual Ability Test

General Chemistry

Organic Chemistry

General Biology

Quantitative Analysis

Reading Comprehension

Perceptual Ability Test

You maybe skimming the list and have seen everything there aforementioned before: Chemistry, Organic Chemistry, and Quantitative Analysis. Then you come across *Perceptual Ability Test*. You may have not heard of this before and wonder what it is.

The PAT or Perceptual Ability Test is a critical component of the DAT since this is a subject lots of students never have seen before. While some people find this section to be fun and relaxing, others struggle through it. The PAT is unlike any other section; it is designed to test how well you can visualize and perform spatial problems in your head. Unlike the other sections which you took classes for, many people didn't complete a class that taught you how to visualize or rotate objects in your mind. For some, it comes naturally. For others, it's a skill that has to be learned. Why would the writers of the DAT put such a tricky section on the test? Since dentists work in very difficult and small spaces, the use of small mouth mirrors is necessary. Also, dentists constantly rely on radiographs of teeth to see cavities and other pathology. Radiographs are given in a two dimensional manner and you have to mentally form a three dimensional image. Now you can understand why this portion of the DAT is very important and relative to dental school. This part also gives the admission committee a clue if you have the capabilities of visualizing mentally 2-D images and making them 3-D images in your head.

There are six sections on the PAT and each type of problem tests different aspects of visualization. If you are appropriately prepared, this part can be the most entertaining. As a dentist you will be performing procedures in tight spaces, and upside down using only a hand mirror. In the beginning it seems to be a very daunting task, making you a little loopy at times. However, with practice, you will be perfect at it. Personally, this was my favorite section on the DAT. Compared to other sections, the PAT required me to use other skills and nicely broke up the academic portion of the test. The key to doing well on the PAT is practice. To do this, many people start working with their hands to improve hand-eye coordination (whether its playing with Lego's, building model toys, or painting). The PAT tends to be a "love it" or "hate it" section. However, the more you practice the better you will do!

Examples of PAT problems:

These PAT problem examples were donated by www.datpat.com, an independent Dental Admission Test Prep Company.

Part I: Keyholes

For questions 1 through 15:

For every question in this part, a 3D object will be displayed at the left. The figure on the left is followed by five openings or apertures all labeled A-E.

The goal is the same for each question. Imagine how the object at the left looks from all directions, not only that is shown. Choose one of the five apertures presented which would allow the object to pass through if the proper side were inserted first. Select the appropriate letter and continue onwards.

Keep in Mind:

    You can rotate the 3D object in any way. It is possible to insert the object via a side that is not shown through the aperture.

    Once the 3D object has started going through the aperture, it may not be rotated or turned in any way. The object must pass completely through the aperture in the condition it is pushed in.

The scale of the 3D object and aperture are the same scale.

No irregularities in any unseen part of the 3D object.

Only one correct answer is represented for each object.

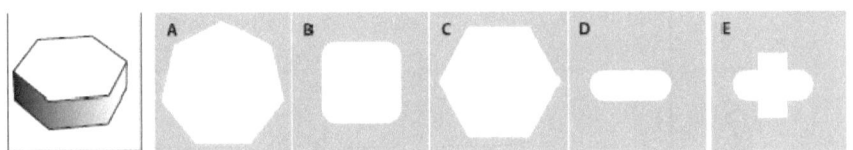

CHOICES:

a) A   ♦   b) B   ♦   c) C   ♦   d) D   ♦   e) E

Answer: C

Part II:

For Questions 16 – 30:

Here are presented top, front, and end views of various objects. All views are presented without perspective. Points in the viewed surface are presented along parallel lines of sight.

TOP VIEW: looking down on the object

FRONT VIEW: view of object from the front

END VIEW: lateral view of the object

Lines that cannot be seen in certain perspectives are represented by dotted lines.

You are given two views of a particular object and it is the goal to find the missing view from the four choices given.

Example:

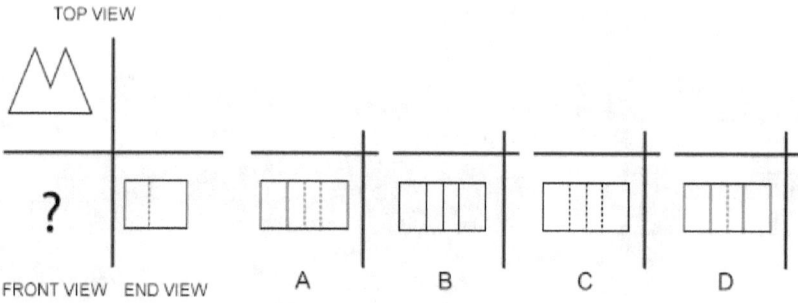

Answer: C.

Part III: Angle Ranking

For Questions 31 – 45:

Each question in this section shows for INTERIOR angles, labeled 1 through 4. Examine the four interior angles presented in each question.

Rank each question's angles in order from the smallest to largest. Select the answer choice that represents the correct ranking.

Example:

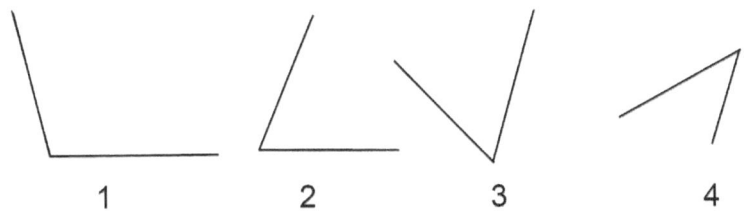

1   2   3   4

CHOICES:

a) 4-3-2-1

b) 3-1-2-4

c) 3-4-1-2

d) 1-3-4-2

Answer: A

Part IV: Hole Punching

For questions 46 – 60:

In these questions, a flat, square piece of paper is folded on or more times. Dotted lines indicate the original position of the paper, and the solid lines indicate the position of the actual folded paper. The folded paper remains within the boundaries of the original, flat sheet. The paper is not turned or twisted. There are one, two, or three folds per question.

Once the final fold is performed, one or more holes are punched in the paper. Once the hole(s) is (are) punched, mentally unfold the paper and ascertain the position(s) of the hole(s) on the original flat sheet.

Select the answer choice that represents the same pattern of dark circles that would reflect the position of holes on the unfolded sheet. There is only one correct pattern for each question.

Example:

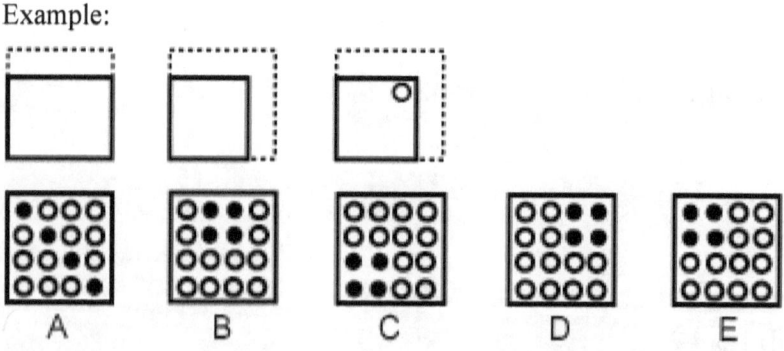

Answer: D

Part V: Cube Counting

For questions 61-75:

Each figure presented in this section has been constructed by cementing together identical cubes. After being cemented, each figure was varnished on all sides EXCEPT for the bottom (where the figure rests). The only hidden cubes are the ones that are necessary to support other cubes in the figure.

Examine each figure carefully regarding the number of sides on each cube that have been varnished. The following questions ask for this information. Select the correct answer choice from the ones provided. **NOTE: 0 is not a correct answer to any question and one figure will be used for multiple questions.**

FIGURE C

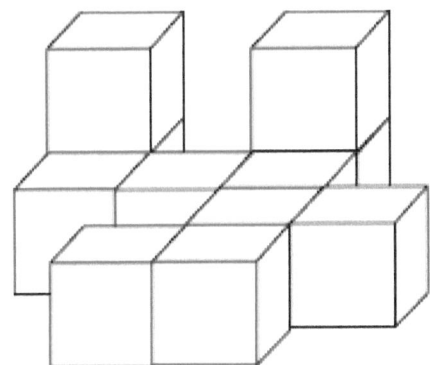

In Figure C, how many cubes have five of their exposed sides painted?

a) 1 cube

b) 2 cubes

c) 3 cubes

d) 4 cubes

e) 5 cubes

Answer: B

Part VI: Paper Folding

For questions 76 through 90.

In the following questions, a flat pattern is presented. This pattern will be folded into a 3D figure; the correct 3D figure is one of the four answer choices illustrated to the right of the unfolded pattern. There is only one correct 3D figure for each question. The pattern at the left represents the outside of the figure.

Example:

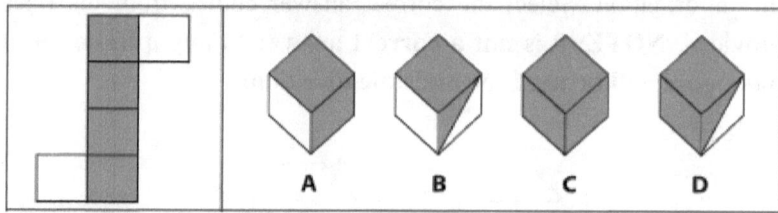

CHOICES:

a) A

b) B

c) C

d) D

Answer: A

~~~
ಸಾ ಣ
~~~

The key to doing well on the DAT/PAT is to study, study, and study some more! How long should you study? I've known people who prepared for three months studying a few hours a day and others who studied for 10 hours a day for a month. Personally, I prepared on my own studying a few hours a day for a couple of months. As I said before, the more you see the information the easier it will be. And the more you study, the easier it is to recall the information.

Obviously, you want to take the prerequisites first then study for this exam to have the full knowledge of all the subjects. You may notice that physics is not on this test, but it is a prerequisite for dental school. So if you want to take this test sooner than later you may want to take the required subjects first.

Now let's go over the subjects on the DAT in detail.

The goal of this section is to see what you retained or understood of your basic core prerequisite classes including Biology, Chemistry, and Organic Chemistry. Biology seems to be a section many students struggle with since the questions are quite varied. The test makers throw weird facts and questions which they can get from anywhere. The best approach is to use the syllabus given by the ADA and systematically go over each subject thoroughly. Organization is the key for these subjects since what the DAT may ask you maybe a small tidbit you learned in class or never learned at all. However, utilizing a good review book will be very important. Once this section is reviewed I will go over some effective test preparation strategies, especially for the DAT exam. Here are the sections on the DAT:

SECTION	Total amount of time allotted	Number of questions	Time to answer each question
Natural Sciences	90 min	100	54 seconds
Perceptual Ability	60 min	90	40.2 seconds
Reading Comprehension	60 min	50	72 seconds
Quantitative Reasoning	45 min	40	67.8 seconds

Based on the syllabus given by the American Dental Association (ADA) who writes the DAT, here is what you can expect for the dental admission test:

Survey of the Natural Sciences
Biology Content Specifications

40 items

I. Cell and Molecular Biology

    A. Origin of Life

    B. Cell metabolism (including photosynthesis)/Enzymes

    C. Cellular Processes

    D. Thermodynamics

    E. Organelle structure and function

    F. Mitosis/Meiosis

    G. Cell structure

    H. Experimental cell biology

II. Diversity of Life: Biological Organization and Relationship of Major Taxa (Five-Kingdom System)

    A. Monera

    B. Plantae

    C. Animalia

    D. Protista

    E. Fungi

    F. Anything else that you may learn during botany and animal physiology

III. Vertebrate Anatomy and Physiology: Structure and Function of Systems

    A. Integumentary System

    B. Skeletal System

    C. Muscular System

    D. Circulatory System

    E. Immunological System

    F. Digestive System

    G. Respiratory System

    H. Urinary System

    I. Nervous System (including sense organs)

    J. Endocrine System

    K. Reproductive System

IV. Developmental Biology

    A. Fertilization

    B. Descriptive embryology

    C. Developmental mechanisms

    D. Experimental embryology

V. Genetics

    A. Molecular genetics

    B. Human genetics

    C. Classical genetics

    D. Chromosomal genetics

    E. Genetic technology

VI. Evolution, Ecology, and Behavior

    A. Natural Selection

    B. Population genetics/Speciation

    C. Population and community ecology

    D. Ecosystem

Survey of the Natural Sciences
General Chemistry Content Specifications

30 items

I. Stoichiometry and General Concepts

- A. Percent composition.
- B. Empirical formulae
- C. Balancing equations
- D. Moles and molecular formulas
- E. Molar mass
- F. Density
- G. Calculations from balanced equations

II. Gases
- A. Kinetic molecular theory of gases
- B. Dalton's gas law
- C. Boyle's gas law
- D. Charles's gas law
- E. Ideal gas law

III. Liquids and Solids
- A. Intermolecular forces
- B. Phase changes
- C. Vapor pressure
- D. Structures
- E. Polarity
- F. Properties

IV. Solutions
- A. Polarity
- B. Properties
    1. Colligative
    2. Non-colligative
- C. Forces
- D. Concentration calculations

V. Acids and Bases
- A. pH
- B. Strength
- C. Brønsted-Lowry reactions
- D. Calculations

VI. Chemical Equilibria
- A. Molecular
- B. Acid/base
- C. Precipitation
- D. Calculations
- E. Le Chatelier's principle

VII. Thermodynamics and Thermochemistry
- A. Laws of thermodynamics
- B. Hess's law
- C. Spontaneity
- D. Enthalpies and entropies
- E. Heat transfer

VIII. Chemical Kinetics
- A. Rate Laws
- B. Activation Energy
- C. Half-life

IX. Oxidation-Reduction Reactions
- A. Balancing equations
- B. Determination of oxidation numbers
- C. Electrochemical calculations
- D. Electrochemical concepts and terminology

X. Atomic and Molecular Structure
- A. Electron configuration

    B. Orbital types

    C. Lewis-Dot diagrams

    D. Atomic theory

    E. Quantum theory

    F. Molecular geometry

    G. Bond types

    H. Sub-atomic particles

XI. Periodic Properties

    A. Representative elements

    B. Transition elements

    C. Periodic trends

    D. Descriptive chemistry

XII. Nuclear Reactions

    A. Balancing equations

    B. Binding energy

    C. Decay processes

    D. Particles

    E. Terminology

XIII. Laboratory

    A. Basic Techniques

    B. Equipment

    C. Error analysis

    D. Safety

Survey of the Natural Sciences
Organic Chemistry Content Specifications

30 items

I. Mechanisms: Reactions

    A. SN1

    B. SN2

    C. Elimination

    D. Addition

    E. Free radical

    F. Substitution mechanisms

II. Chemical and Physical Properties of Molecules and Organic Analysis

    A. Inter- and intra-molecular forces

    B. Separation

    C. Introductory infrared spectroscopy

    D. 1HNMR spectroscopy

    E. 13CNMR

    F. Chemical identification

    G. Stability

    H. Solubility

    I. Polarity

III. Stereochemistry

    A. Conformational analysis

    B. Geometric isomers

"Give me six hours to chop down a tree and I will spend four sharpening the axe." (Abraham Lincoln)

ಸಃ ಣ

There have been many hours spent at the library, coffee shops, even online forums where students ask, "What's the best way to prepare for the DAT?" No matter how many times someone asks this question, the answer always stays the same. The more work you do, the better you will do. Regardless, there is a multitude of information you learn in your undergraduate courses and it's not fair to assume that the DAT covers all of it. You need to understand the depth of the DAT first then recognize the major topics that the test makers want you know and understand. Once you have the map figured out and know where you are going, you can finally utilize resources from your classes, including your text books, notes, and other supplemental materials.

First of all, go through the material. Look at all the sections and see what's covered. Next, be sure to study the sections you think you know super well. You won't be wasting time reading information you know, because refreshing yourself will reinforce the concepts even more so you are prepared even more for the DAT. That being said, don't spend all your time reading the parts you know. Go through everything and spend time on the sections you have trouble with. As rudimentary as this may sound, students like to study sections they already know fairly well but anything that seems foreign or hard to them they want to skim or skip. The reason is that it helps build their confidence while they are studying, but when they take the test they don't score as well as they expected because they neglected the subjects that needed their attention the most. This is a fact of life; people are just more comfortable studying information they know and got an A in, but not what they got a C in. However, for this exam it is important to focus on your weaknesses then on your strengths. We will discuss test strategies later during the exam. In addition to studying out of books, take practice tests. This will help you become familiar with how the questions are phrased, and will show you where you need to focus when you are studying. Another thing that can help you for the DAT is to also see why you got an answer wrong. If the explanation doesn't make sense or isn't explained well, you can always consult other texts and people. While studying for the Organic Chemistry section of the DAT, I constantly found myself needing help. I could see how the mechanisms worked, but the question I had was "WHY?" After consulting my old textbooks, notes, exams, and still not understanding the problems, I went back to my old chemistry professor and got help. You need to study *actively* instead of *passively*.

Your Study Environment

What is the difference between active preparation versus passive preparation? In order to study actively, your study environment is key. First and foremost, your study environment should be comfortable and clean. Extra stuff you do not need around you while studying is a problem. Having pictures, the television on, or other unrelated material around you while studying is going to deter you from studying effectively. I want you to ask yourself how you studied for a certain class that you did well in? Everyone has different techniques and this is no way to tell you how to study. I know for some classes like mathematics, I used to study with my iPod on. Other classes such as Organic Chemistry, I needed everything to be quiet. This chapter will cover some standardized test study techniques which worked not only for me, but for many of my colleagues in dental school.

Environment

This can be in your room, at the library, or at a coffee shop. Regardless where it is it needs to be organized and the study material should be organized in a manner it can be reviewed easily. Organize your materials effectively for each subject that you are studying. Once I got all of my materials and notes, I used the syllabus for the exam and organized all of my textbooks, notes, etc. I would have them organized at all times in case I felt like taking them out to a coffee shop or library. Remember, disorganization is the main ingredient to procrastination. When your materials are ready to go, so are you.

Study Schedule

Like I mentioned before, there are many ways to study for the DAT. The best method is to pay attention in your college classes and take detailed and well organized notes. However, by the time most of us are ready to take the DAT we have thrown out our class notes, sold our books back, and completely erased those classes from our memory. If this is you, do not panic. If you paid attention in class, which I am sure you did, and scored reasonably well on exams, you probably can start recalling quite effortlessly as you start preparing for the DAT.

Let's look at study strategies. First, look at the allotted time you have. Some people spend six months to prepare for the DAT, but most people will spend about two to three months, roughly. Each person is different and each individual's time constraints are different. I know many students who took a quarter or semester off to study for it, however this is not advisable unless you are on time to graduate. Studying from spring to early summer is probably the best time. Also, when you study for the DAT, it would be advisable to take a lighter course load than what you are customary to. For example, if you have outstanding electives for your major, it may be a good idea to couple them with your DAT studying.

I have seen many people study for the DAT in conjunction with DAT subject classes such as organic chemistry, but many of those students felt they were overly stressed while studying for both. Do yourself a favor and keep your schedule light. This also means keep your work schedule light as well. These concepts may seem mundane, but they are very important not only for studying for the DAT, but also for your future exams in and out of dental school.

I recommend taking about 6-8 weeks to study. If you take to long to prepare, then you may start forgetting the material you first started studying. If you are taking six months to prepare for this exam, what are the chances you will still have the material you studied in week one still fresh in your head?

Here is my approach:

First and foremost, register for the DAT test. Pick a date that is comfortable for you – one that is not rushed. Based on the date you picked and your current class/work load, you will have an end goal. This is very important. One of the benefits of the DAT is that you can take it any time of the year. However, this can be a disadvantage when you do not know when you are taking the test. Having a theoretical date is not a good idea since mentally you will keep pushing the date back when delays happen in your studies. So take the next step, and register online at the American Dental Association's website.

While the study materials only come in books, the actual DAT is given on a computer and is timed per section. Many people have said reading on a computer proved to be a problem, but it can easily be overcome. A simple solution: read the daily news online. Whether it is the *New York Times* or a celebrity gossip column, the more you read, the more comfortable reading on the computer will be. Granted, the more complicated the reading material, the more of an improvement you will see on the reading section. The articles presented on the DAT are simple scientific articles. The questions are based on those articles and are comprehension based. An average reading comprehension passage is up to 1,500 words with about 20 or so questions.

Quantitative Analysis is the last portion of the DAT. This section is mathematics. Many students feel they are the most pressured for time in this section of the exam. There are many reasons for this, one being that this section probably requires the most analytical ability on the test. Since this is the last section, by the time you get to this section you are pretty mentally burned out. However, the questions on this section are not made to trick you. You just need to understand the types of problems the DAT likes to test. The core subjects on this section are basic statistics, fractions, probability questions, and word problems. There will be some pre-calculus, but nothing too daunting.

From this section you should take the following:

- Work in an organized environment without distractions.
- Register for the DAT so you have a date set.
- Understand the basic components of the exam.

Now that you've seen the basics of the test, your next step is to set up a schedule that will help you study successfully.

Here are several sample schedules that many of my colleagues used.

Sample One:
Study time: 6 weeks

Method of studying: class notes, Kaplan DAT book, and sample exams

    Week One: Biology

    Week Two: Chemistry/Organic Chemistry

    Week Three: Organic Chemistry

    Week Four: PAT and Quantitative Ability

    Week Five: Sample exams

    Week Six: Sample exams

This student scored 21 Academic and 20 PAT. He applied to 14 schools, got 10 interviews, went on four interviews and got accepted to all four schools. His GPA was 3.5 average and 3.4 science. His major was Zoology.

Sample Two:
Study time 8 weeks

This student used the day of the week method. Each day, he would study for two to three hours on an individual subject.

    Monday: Biology

Tuesday: Chemistry

Wednesday: Organic Chemistry

Thursday: PAT

Friday: Quantitative Ability

Saturday: Reading Comprehension

Sunday: Review subjects, study sample exams

This student got a 22 Academic score and 19 PAT score. He applied to six schools, got three interviews, and got accepted to all three schools. His GPA was 3.6 and his Science GPA was 3.2. His major was Sociology.

Sample Three:

In this sample, the student felt very comfortable with General Chemistry and Organic Chemistry (he was a Biochemistry major). He decided to take a risk and focus only on a few subjects, and spent four weeks studying. He also took a review course which he said gave him an outline of the structure of the exam.

Week One: Biology, Reading Comprehension, and Quantitative Ability

Week Two: Biology, Reading Comprehension, and Quantitative Ability

Week Three: PAT

Week Four: PAT and sample exams

This student got a 19 Academic score 20 PAT score. His GPA was 3.3 and his Science GPA was 3.5. He applied to seven schools, got five interviews, and went to four interviews. He got accepted to one school.

Sample Four:

This last student spent four months preparing. Initially, she wanted to take the exam in two months but kept changing the date. Her major was Biology with a minor in Communications. Her schedule was random and she studied using her class notes and sample exams. In retrospect, she wished her organization was better and that she would have followed the examples of the students above. Her major was biology. Her GPA was 3.6 and had a 3.2 Science GPA. Her DAT score was 19 Academic and 17 PAT. She applied to 18 schools, got six interviews, and went on all six interviews. She was accepted to three schools.

All four of the examples above were successful in achieving admission to dental school. Each of the samples used a different method of studying. You may tailor your schedule to one of the above examples and adjust it to your needs. In my survey of more than 50 students, the times of studying varied from one week to over nine months. The average study time was around two to three months. Each student stated that it was imperative to schedule the test first so you have a set goal to take the exam. Some of the people who took over four months said one of the main reasons they studied so long was because they did not have a definite set date for the exam. Due to not having this "pressure," they kept studying extra without taking the exam. This is one of the caveats of having a test that can be taken on any day of the year. It is a hindrance to your study schedule and your application schedule.

A few years back, a test taker could change the test date as many times as possible as long as it was done two business days prior. Today, there is a fee each time the exam date is changed. It is best not to change the test date, as it makes it easier for you to do it again. This is one thing about standardized tests: no matter how much or how long you prepare, you never feel fully prepared. I have asked people with impeccable grade point averages and high DAT scores if they felt fully prepared and everyone said no. So do not get caught up in changing your exam over and over again. The best strategy is to set a date that you are comfortable with and then go for it.

First and foremost, look at the DAT syllabus and see what areas you may have problems. Make a rough outline of your study schedule. Be reasonable. If you think you can study for 12 hours a day for one month, you may regret it and lose confidence if you can't meet that objective. Know your limitations. By now after spending countless hours studying, taking classes, balancing your social life, work, and school, you'll likely to have a good idea of what your study habits are. Utilize that knowledge and make a realistic and reasonable study schedule. It may be you know for a fact you are unable to study for longer than three hours a day. Then set yourself three hours a day for however many days that you need to feel comfortable with the exam. Typically, if you set aside three hours a day for six days you should be in good shape, especially if you give yourself about six to eight weeks to prepare for the exam. Once you know that for the next two months you can devote a certain time to focus on the DAT, schedule the DAT exam. You can choose to organize your schedule weekly or daily as the example students.

Here is a simple table of how long you should prepare. Obviously, you are the best judge for yourself – it all depends on your confidence level. If you paid attention in class, did well on exams, and kept your notes organized, then you will need less preparation time. If you took your core subjects two years ago, threw away all your notes, and did average on your exams, then you will need more time to study.

- Comfortable with all materials: four to six weeks prep time
- Comfortable with four out of six areas: six to eight weeks prep time
- Uncomfortable with all areas: eight to 10 weeks prep time
- Forgotten all areas, not comfortable with any subject areas: 12-14 weeks prep time

Now look at the above averages. I added two additional weeks to the averages I got from my surveys. This accounts for vacations, school tests, and illnesses, all which may add additional time to the preparation time.

It is obvious that those who did well in their classes spent less time preparing for the test. The average was about four weeks for these individuals. Most of these individuals had above a 3.5 GPA average. The second group generally spent up to a month and a half preparing, were all good students, but had that occasional B- or C in a core class and spent a few weeks additional on patching up their weakness. This group had an average GPA of 3.4. The third group either was taking the DAT with a long break between their core classes, or simply decided to throw their knowledge away after their classes. This group had an average GPA of 3.2. The majority of this group said that the length of time between the subjects and the DAT made them uneasy with the subject material. The second reasoning was they just did not do as well in these subjects. The subjects that these students felt the most uneasy about were chemistry and organic chemistry. The fourth group who took over three months to prepare, had many reasons. One reason was not selecting a concrete test date before they began studying. Second, this group was disorganized and they did not have a plan of attack prior to the study sessions. This group's GPA was varied between 3.0 and 3.7. The above summary of the survey is to show you that there are several common things that the first two groups had.

Chart of importance:

Test date was determined before studying

Student had an organized study schedule

Student took the DAT close to finishing their core classes

All of the above considerations must be taken into account prior to studying for this test.

Once you get comfortable with the subject matter, you will need to take some practice exams. I recommend taking "simulation" exams and time yourself just like you are taking the real exam. Many software titles and books are available for this purpose.

Once the test is completed:

Once you have completed the DAT, you should have a sense of relief. The beauty of this exam is that you get your scores right away. There is no waiting period. Now let's strategize on how the DAT is graded and what is a competitive score.

The DAT consists of two main scores. One is the Academic Score and the PAT Score. These are the scores that most schools look at. The Academic Score consists of an average of all of the subjects, minus the PAT portion of the exam. A competitive Academic Score is around 20 and a 19 for PAT.

GPA	Min Academic Score	Minimum PAT Score
4.0	18	17
3.9	18	17
3.8	18	17
3.7	19	18
3.6	19	18
3.5	20	18
3.4	20	19
3.3	20	20
3.2	21	21
3.1	21	21
3.0	21	21
<2.9	22	21

This table is a general outline on average GPA, minimum Academic Score, and the PAT Score, all which are needed to be considered competitive for majority of the dental schools in the United States. Obviously, there are other factors such as volunteering and life experience, but the "meat and potatoes" of your application are the numbers: GPA and DAT scores. As you can see, the lower the GPA, the higher the scores are needed to maintain competitiveness. The majority of schools have a cut-off GPA of 3.0. That means if you have a GPA of lower than 3.0 then your applications may not even be reviewed by the admission committee. You have to understand that the first step of the application process is usually done by computer. You send your application to a processing department called the AADSAS in Washington, D.C. which is run by ADEA. They input your numbers and send off your application to the dental schools. Here at the dental school, based on certain numerical cut-offs, your application is screened further once you meet the basic numbers (in this case GPA and DAT scores). After meeting the first cut-off, the admissions committee will look closer at your application and may send you a secondary application for further information. Usually the secondary application requires you to give more detailed information, mainly through essays.

After receiving your secondary application and approving your GPA and DAT scores, you might be granted an interview. When there are several thousand applicants for about 100 or so spots in most schools, the competition is very rigorous.

Since the grading of the exam is immediate, you either will be happy or very upset that same day. Let's say your GPA is 3.2 and you get a score of 17 academic and 16 PAT score. Here, you know that you are not at the cut-off from the chart above. It would be recommended to register again for the DAT. The ADA recommends at least 90 days between your DAT test dates. This is done for several reasons. One is that the testing board wants you to study hard for the second time around. Another reason is that since you have already taken the DAT, you may remember questions. Every 30-90 days new questions are added to the databank. There are many versions of the test so it is not a great idea to only study stuff you remembered during the exam. You may want to remember certain topics which you had difficulty with during the exam and focus on those to improve your score.

If you do need to retake the DAT you can still submit your application and write to the Dean of Admissions letting them know you are retaking the DAT. It may delay your application just a little bit, but if you have strategized and organized well, then it should not hinder your chance of matriculating into dental school. We will talk more about organizing your application and preparing for the worst in the next section.

ଚ୍ଛ ଗ୍ଧ

THE DENTAL APPLICATION

The dental application is a process. There are several parts to the application which are summarized below:

- GPA with transcript
- At least three letters of recommendation
- Application essay
- DAT Scores

The above summarizes the basic ingredients for your application. Dental schools need the above requirements to either send you a secondary and/or interview you. It would be in your best interest to get these as soon as possible so there is no hindrance to your application.

The letters of recommendation need to be from professors, mentors, research professors, as well as working professionals who know you well. If you go to a university where classes are quite large (let's say over 500 students), then it might be more difficult to get good letters of recommendation. It will be necessary to register in a class which is smaller in order for the professor to get to know you better. Before asking for a letter of recommendation you will need to organize a résumé. Ask the person you are interested in obtaining a letter from if they would be able to write you a good and beneficial letter. It is better to get an honest "no" than an average or mediocre letter from them. Since you are the one applying to dental school you need to have these letters prior to application. You must give ample time for your professors to complete the letter. A good amount of time is four to six weeks. Also, follow up with your professor and make sure they know how urgent it is. Sometimes, professors get swamped or they simply forget, so reminding them is a good idea. This applies to any boss you may have, as well as a dental mentor. Ideally, you should have three good letters of recommendation which highlight more than your grade in a class. It would be good to get a letter from a science professor, a non-science professor, and someone who knows your passion for dentistry. Here is a table for letter of recommendations you may want to consider.

Science Professor	Non-Science Professor	Other
Organic Chemistry	English	Dentist
Biology	History	Work related
General Chemistry	Language	Pastor
Genetics	Music	Volunteer location
Biochemistry	Anthropology	Dental resident
Research Lab	Communications	Dental Specialist
Microbiology	Math	Teacher Assistant

The above table is a sample list of recommendations. You can ask whomever you choose but you must make sure that they are able to write a powerful recommendation for you. It defeats the purpose if the professor hardly knows you. For this reason, it might be better to ask a professor from an upper level science class where there is a better professor-student interaction. A non-science professor may be an interesting class you took such as music or language.

Submitting your application:

Once your application is ready to be submitted, it will be first sent to AADSAS which is a branch of the ADEA. Although most schools participate in AADSAS, not every school does. This needs to be verified with AADSAS and the prospective school. Here the application and its information are compiled and organized for each of the dental schools you have applied to. This information is packaged and sent to the schools, who then process and begin their screening process. Once they screen your application they may send you a secondary application which entails more questions. There are several reasons for secondary applications, and some of these include:

- Getting more thorough answers to certain questions
- Seeing if you are still interested in the school
- Collect more money.

Once a school receives your secondary application, it may offer you an interview. For most schools interviewing, this begins in early September of the year before matriculation. For example, if you want to enter dental school in the spring of 2012, the school may start interviewing as early as September of 2011. Receiving an interview is a milestone of the application process, for it shows the applicant that the school is seriously considering you for admission.

୧୦ ଔ

To reiterate the application process:

A. Complete College Core Prerequisites

    Biology, one year

    General Chemistry, one year

    Organic Chemistry, one year

    Calculus/Statistics, half year

    English, half year

    Microbiology, half year

    Biochemistry, half year

B) Dental Admission Test

C) Application Essay

D) Letters of Recommendation

E) Transcript

    Once the above steps are finished, your primary application process is complete. Next you may encounter the following:

A) Secondary Application

B) Interview

Basic Information about AADSAS and the application:

Acronym: Associated American Dental Schools Application Service (AADSAS)

Administered by American Dental Education Association (ADEA)

Access AADSAS thru the ADEA site: www.adea.org

Texas Schools require additional application information

It may take about 10 to 12 hours to complete the entire application, so make sure to have all papers and information handy and a stable internet connection.

The AADSAS application is usually available from mid-May on, every year.

Prepare for all sections before you apply.

Apply early, ideally before June 15th, even if you have not taken the DAT or completed all the prerequisites.

Customer Service

Mon thru Fri 9:00am – 4:30pm (Eastern)

Call (800) 353-2237 or (202) 289-7201 and expect to wait on hold

E-mail: csraadsas@adea.org It's usually best to avoid e-mail since response time is longer.

Completing the Application Outline:

Menus: Get familiar with all of the buttons and pages of the application

Section 1: Biographical Info

Section 2: Parent and Family Information

Section 3: Secondary School Information

Section 4: Colleges Attended
- Send Transcripts as soon as AADSAS is submitted
- Use provided Transcript Matching Form

Section 5: Coursework
- Update all of the transcripts of each college you attended.
- Be sure to enter classes currently "currently enrolled/in progress" and future planned classes.
- Know that your college GPA and what AADSAS converts may vary. This is the true for schools that have grades on the point system instead of the letter grade system.

Section 6: DAT Scores
- Schools require the official score report from the ADA for your DAT.
- If you have not taken the DAT, you can state a future prospective date. Make sure you let the admissions officer know that you have not taken the DAT.

Section 7: Dentistry Experience
- Make sure you have some experience in a dental setting. 100 hours is ideal.
- Keep a log sheet.

Section 8: Letters of Recommendation
- Schools have varying requirements for Letters of Recommendation. (LOR's)
- Use provided LOR Matching Form.
- Talk to prospective LOR contributors and give them enough time.
- Organize and give your LOR contributors everything from résumé, essays, or anything else you want them to write about you.

- Make sure to waive your right to see letter or recommendation so schools do not think you are sending only the best ones.

Section 9: Extracurricular/Volunteer/Community Service
- Schools really want to see significant community involvement.
- Track these well as you volunteer so you can complete this section.

Section 10: Work Experience

Section 11: Research Experience

Section 12: Background Information
- This includes manual dexterity experience.
- Talk about dental experience, and other hobbies that use your hands.

Section 13: Personal Statement
- This is your chance to point out your strengths.
- Prepare this before May 15th.
- Have professors and colleagues review and edit your statement.

Section 14: Release Statements

Section 15: Awards, Honors, Scholarships
- Include everything from high school on.

Section 16: Dental School Designations
- Make sure to review the application many times for any errors, especially spelling errors.

ಎ ಆ

After Submitting the Application

- ✓ Keep tabs by calling AADSAS every week. Make sure your application goes through and all the materials are sent.
- ✓ Check the supplemental materials page constantly and make sure everything is taken care of.
- ✓ Check the school site for supplementary information/ applications. Some schools do have them on their site and it can make your application go much faster if you complete it right away.
- ✓ Once completed, the entire application can take up to eight weeks to process.
- ✓ After three weeks, call all schools to follow-up until you get the confirmation from every school that your file is 100% complete.
- ✓ Understand that AADSAS can lose information, so be patient and ready if they ask you to resend something you already have sent. Keep extra copies of transcripts handy.
- ✓ Call the schools and see if they are receiving the information from AADSAS.

⁂

THE DENTAL ESSAY: YOUR SELF PORTRAIT

One of the most critical parts of the application is the dental essay. Here you have an opportunity to write about yourself and why you are choosing the field of dentistry. In this chapter we will break down several questions and brainstorm ideas for your dental essay. Below are a few questions that will get your mind ready not only for interviews but for your essay. Your essay is a concise written expression of why you are choosing the field of dentistry. The more brainstorming you do the better. It will also make your essay become more powerful. Answer each question in a few sentences.

What is unique about you culturally? Tell us about your upbringing?

_____
_____
_____

What is unique about you academically? Why did you pick your major? What interesting classes did you take during college?

_____
_____
_____

What is unique about you socially? Do you do anything unique outside of work and school? What are your hobbies?

_____
_____
_____

What is unique about you in general? What is something only a few people know about you?

_____
_____
_____

Why did you choose dentistry? Was there anything that pushed your interest toward dentistry?

_____
_____
_____

What is your experience with dentistry? Volunteering? Observing?

_____
_____
_____

What things do you like about dentistry?

_____
_____
_____

What things do you not like about dentistry?

_____
_____
_____

Have you done research? If so, briefly explain what you researched? Did you get published?

_____
_____
_____

Do you play sports?

_____
_____
_____

Have you won any awards or recognition for your achievements?

_____
_____
_____
_____

Once you have completed the above questions you are well on your way to writing your dental essay. You can use the information above and organize your thoughts on how you want to proceed with your essay. These are also some frequent questions that many dental schools ask during their interviews. Also, if you complete the above questions, you can type up your responses and give them to those people you are requesting letters of recommendation from. It will help them get to you know you better and will help them use the information you provided to build a powerful letter of recommendation.

ഇ ൡ

Sample Admission Essays

The following four sample essays were taken from successful applicants. Each of these applicants came from different backgrounds and was successfully admitted to dental school. Personal information has been omitted to protect the privacy of the candidates. As you read these samples, think of ways you can implement similar ideas based on your personal life and background.

Sample Essay #1

It might confuse you as to why I, a MBA student, am applying to dental school. My mother and father, both businessmen, have been in business for the last 30 years. They raised me to be an entrepreneur who would someday take over what they had started. Since I was 15 years old, I have helped my parents to organize and manage our business. I grew up believing that this was what I wanted. However, my interest in dentistry soon dominated my ambitions.

As a child, I could not wait for my bi-annual visit to the dentist. I always loved the free gifts: the toothbrush, the mouthwash, and the toys. I loved the array of instruments that the dentist had laid out. As the years went on, I volunteered at different dental practices. One summer, I volunteered at [Kool Dental Smiles], a practice owned by Dr. [John Doe]. I love the friendly environment, the patients, and Dr. [John Doe]'s willingness to show me how he diagnoses and treats patients. Through these experiences, I was able to see what a career in dentistry really entails. By the time I was a junior in high school, my interest in dentistry evolved from a childish curiosity to a profession I wanted to pursue. But how could I become a dentist? It was already decided that I was going to take over my parent's business and fulfill the dream they had for me.

In the fall of 2002, I entered [Beta University], majoring in business. Soon after my classes started, I began to question whether I had made the right decision. There wasn't anything in my business classes that intrigued me. I obtained an internship at the [organization] in New York City in the summer after my sophomore year. I hoped this would help me to further explore the business world. Working at [organization] was an invaluable experience. It allowed me to see a different aspect of business. Most importantly, however, I learned that business was not satisfying to me and a career in this path was not something I wanted do for the rest of my life.

A major turning point in my life came on New Year's Day 2001, the day I decided I was going to be a dentist. On this day, my father had a stroke. The doctor said that he may not be able to walk or speak again. The thought of losing my father was unbearably painful. My father had told me before that if something had happened to him then I would be in charge of the family business. He was putting me in charge of what he worked so many years to create. The idea of my running his business was becoming a reality, and this was my chance to give back to my family.

The doctor who helped my father soon interrupted us during our time at the hospital and I remember looking at him with such reverence, for he held the fate of my entire family in his hands. Because of that doctor's knowledge and empathy, my father is in good health now. He did not just save my father's life or relieve my father from pain; he helped my entire family and relieved all of us from pain. I never appreciated the importance of helping another individual until I was the one being helped.

My father's stroke brought me face to face with the conflict between my obligation to the innermost circle, my family, and my desire to help a broader community and beyond. I always believed that following my parent's wishes was my way of making a difference. It was not. I wanted to contribute to others, not just to my family. The circle within which I wanted to make a difference widened. I cannot imagine there being anything more satisfying or rewarding than helping a person in need. I knew right then that my aspiration to pursue a career in dentistry would allow me to achieve that goal.

Becoming a dentist is not simply fulfilling a childhood ambition; it is my way to improve the lives of others by promoting oral health and helping people with problems such as gum disease or tooth decay. Dentistry will also give me a chance to utilize my degree in business, if someday I choose to open up my own practice. Furthermore, I want to mentor aspiring dentists as Dr. John Doe did for me. As a start, I founded and am President of the Beta University Pre-Dental Society. I have helped pre-dental students gain exposure to the dental field by organizing trips to different dental schools and inviting dentists to share their experiences.

All my experiences thus far have been preparing me as a person and as an adult. I have spent the last few years exploring and challenging my inner and outer self. Finally, I have come to the realization that the person I want to be is the same person I loved to visit as a child – a dentist. I have worked hard to attain a large amount of exposure and I am now ready and capable of achieving my goal and making my dream a reality.

Sample Essay #2

From an early childhood, my parents instilled in me the values of honesty, self respect, and respect for others. As far back as I can remember, the concept of exploring my curiosities, whether dissecting my toys or building electronic robots, seemed to be infinitely fascinating. My parents continually encouraged me to be active and to explore all that was around me. I surrounded myself with automobile magazines, books, and scientific kits, always looking for new ways to enjoy these things. This happy adolescent environment was interrupted when the reality of war hit home. Under these hostile and many times traumatizing events, my parents made the brave decision to migrate to U.S.A. in the hopes of providing a better future for their children. The experience of war through such innocent eyes could have had a negative impact on the rest of my life. Instead, the horrible event instilled me with a sound understanding of the value of life and a strong desire to develop skills, which would allow me to assist others during times of need.

My academic studies began in the amorphous realm of business management. In the fall of 1998, I decided it was time to sharpen my skills in the marketplace. I gathered associates, raised capital, and launched a business, a private consulting firm offering website design, e-solutions, and graphic design, tailored to the often technologically averse healthcare industry. As President and CEO of this small company, I not only managed my own business, but more importantly I honed my academic skills through real world application. As my education in business progressed, my business career continued to expand, and I soon realized that Internet technology was not what I loved—a difficult conclusion that I reached while busily navigating through the boom times of the Internet. Suddenly, business, as an end unto itself seemed a rather empty proposition. I was unsure of my direction, drifting unfulfilled, looking for a meaningful niche of my own.

In this haze of personal uncertainty, a good friend introduced me to the possibility of working in dentistry. This friend came from a family of dentists and thus was able to reveal a life lived in dentistry. Although the skill set would be wholly different, I would be able to apply much of what I learned through my own endeavors with consulting in the healthcare industry. I knew I needed to spend time in the clinical setting to determine if this is my bliss. I arranged to follow two both of whom patiently explained each procedure, no matter how routine or rudimentary. However, I crossed my own personal crossroad not with such shadowing experiences, which while helpful, served to buttress a budding curiosity about the field of dentistry. It became a pursuit after I was chatting with the doctor as he was literally closing his office and had sent the remainder of his staff home for the evening. A mother came screeching through the parking lot, emerged from her car frantic about how her eight year old son had suffered a dental injury during a sporting activity. Calmly and in a matter of minutes, the doctor alleviated the child's pain and the mother's worry. It could not be any clearer for me than at that particular moment: dentistry was an avenue for me to help people, make a difference in their lives, and build relationships of trust and care. The curriculum shift in order to seriously pursue dentistry as a vocation, I knew, would require a radical change from what I was accustomed to. From starting out not knowing if a mole was really anything more than a feature on "Uncle Henry's" nose, to a serious student of science, to soon thereafter being awarded a position as a teaching assistant, I noted with great enjoyment my progress in the sciences.

In summary, this is an essay about first looking, then finding, and ultimately following your bliss. For many people, this can be a lifelong pursuit. Luckily, I have found my springboard to this end. Starting my studies as a graduate student in the School of Dentistry, I feel, will be the natural complement to the path I have undertaken. As a dedicated individual driven by an evolution of varied experiences, I plan to continue my studies of dentistry beyond my doctorate. I am determined to play an active role in research, keep up with new dental technologies, and promote oral health in the community.

Sample Dental Essay #3

This is an essay about life change. This is an essay about finally realizing what it is you are meant to do, and taking a chance to realize your dreams. This is an essay about my passion to become a dentist.

There are simply no words to describe my fear. A simple bicycle accident had landed me in the doctor's office to receive an occlusion for my badly broken jaw. In addition to the pain, discomfort, and life style restrictions, I was injured psychologically. I felt awkward and indifferent; I was barely able to smile through my disfigured jaw, let alone carry on a conversation. This difficult ordeal left me with a tremendous sense of understanding for oral injuries.

While in the early stages of deciding a career path, I chose to work as a research assistant with a doctor. My work with the doctor introduced me to a wide range of surgical procedures and greatly expanded my interest in the medical sciences. This solidified by decision to pursue a career in the healthcare profession allowing me to help others. To me, this field offered amazing opportunities to really make a difference in this world and help serve my community. I had been introduced early on by family friends to the field of dentistry and had decided to inquire further.

In the natural progression of curiosity, I asked my dentist to allow me to shadow with the goal of gaining an insight to this profession. This shadowing grew to a full time summer volunteer job as his dental assistant. While working alongside him, I witnessed a variety of dental procedures, from the final stages of dental implants to amalgam fillings. In addition to learning much about the technical aspects of dentistry, I developed an appreciation for the care, respect, and personal attention with which the doctor treated every patient. The intrinsic rewards of this profession have stayed with me since and have fueled my passion.

When the experience came to an end, I felt ready to focus all my energy toward learning as much as I could about the field of dentistry. Understanding the academic excellence that the dental profession demanded I geared myself to achieve this. I worked hard at building a reputation of academic excellence balanced with community and peer assisting activities. I thrived by working with others and taking advantage of my open and friendly personality to initiate team work in the learning environment. Realizing the advantages of a group learning environment, a friend and I established the American Student Dental Association Chapter at the university. I became the vice-president of the organization and sought to gain insight of dental specializations, preparation information on the DAT, and application support. I was able through this organization to gain valuable information about dental school and the lifelong pursuit of knowledge within a field. More importantly, I was able to give back to students who were in my shoes several years back.

    The care given to me by medical personnel helped me to develop, at a very young age, a deep interest in helping others. As I grew and became interested in scientific studies, this desire pushed me toward the possibility of a career in dentistry. I was very fortunate to find a mentor willing to indulge my curiosity, and the time spent in the company of cemented my decision to pursue the study of dentistry. It is my personal goal to create an atmosphere of trust and friendship with those in need of my help. It is within this framework that I will serve others the best I can.

    This is an essay about finally realizing what it is you are meant to do, and taking a chance to realize your dreams. This is an essay about my passion to become a dentist. Although the path has not always been as clear as it is now, the closer I move toward actual dentistry, the more confidence I feel in the rightness of my decisions. Now I have direction: I will shine, become the best doctor I can be, and provide the best dental care possible.

Sample Dental Essay #4

Military Academy served as the stepping stone that has shaped in many words my academic discipline and "no quitter" work ethic. This high school had a dynamic student body and the structured curriculum that shaped me in to adulthood. It was during these years in which I realized my passion of working with my hands as a means to hide my speech problems. Anything that kept me physically active seemed to be a solution to my short comings as a speaker.

The next chapter in my life was filled with hard work and challenging times. I was considered an out of state student, forcing me to work and help support my mother and I while paying for tuition and expenses. Even worse, I was confused and scattered in determining what major to pursue. In the fall of 2002, I received my first break allowing me to receive an in-state waiver, saving me thousands. As a result, I was capable of reducing my work hours and focusing more on my studies. A degree in Architecture was the major that I started under, which offered a promising and secure future allowing me to have an interesting and hands on career.

In the summer of 2003, I decided it was time to sharpen my skills in the real world. I applied and was hired as an intern in a consulting firm. This was the first time that I felt accomplished through the usage of my formal education in my work environment. As my work progressed, I learned the importance of helping disadvantaged people and realized the value of making a difference in these areas. As a result, I soon realized that architecture was not what I loved—a difficult conclusion that I reached while busily studying and experiencing the construction industry. Suddenly, architecture was an end unto itself seemed a rather empty proposition. I was unsure of my direction, drifting unfulfilled, looking for a meaningful niche of my own. In this haze of personal uncertainty, I knew what I wanted out of life, which was to make a change by providing a better opportunity for lower income households, but did not know what medium to use.

During these times, a good friend introduced me to the possibility of dentistry. I knew I needed to spend time in the clinical setting to determine if this was a career opportunity for me. I arranged to follow a doctor who patiently explained each procedure to me, no matter how routine or rudimentary.

The curriculum shift needed to seriously pursue dentistry was ambitious to say the least. I knew it would require great effort with no procrastination. As I progressed in this era of change, I encountered the greatest hardship of my life when an incident was brought upon my father. An automobile accident left him with fractured limbs and a broken jaw limiting his daily function at the age of 57. Through the first semester of preparing myself for dental school I scheduled my time in a way so that during the days I would take care of my father and in the evenings I was focusing on classes and studying. My father's accident forced me to become extremely disciplined in time management, and made me realize the real value of life. Experiencing this hardship and seeing my father's struggle through late night pain and being on a liquid diet, I realized the best way to care was through love and knowledge. It was a no-brainer at that point that healthcare givers experience a high level of intrinsic rewards. As a result, I have settled to withstand all challenges in successfully achieving a doctorate in dental Medicine and pursuing a specialty in Oral Surgery. More than ever today we need people to care and love people, and I am ready to do my part in society. I plan on playing an active role in oral health in lower income communities that have traditionally been ignored. I will harness my experiences and my business savvy to make these "untraditional" areas make sense as a practitioner.

The Non-Traditional Applicant

So you realized that your current career path wasn't for you and you decided to enter the dental field. Congratulations! At least now you know what you are passionate about. Based on applicant surveys every year over 25% of the applicant pool belongs to the non-traditional applicant. The following criteria maybe used to differentiate a traditional applicant from a non-traditional applicant:

Traditional Applicant	Non-Traditional Applicant
Applied to dental school right after getting their undergraduate degree.	Had several years of work experience after getting their baccalaureate degree.
Usually minimal life experience other than school.	Possibly married
	Possibly has children
	Went back to school to finish dental school requirements
	Had certain life experiences such as military, business ventures, won the lottery, etc.
	Had a sudden break in their education due to various reasons: sickness, family emergency, etc.
	Traveled abroad for work, etc.

You may utilize the above table to help you explain your unique application in your essay. Schools appreciate students who have different life circumstances. The above information is just some criteria for the non-traditional applicant. The major criterion is that the non-traditional applicant usually has some life experience after graduating with a Bachelor's degree. Some non-traditional students studied in completely different fields and may already have a doctorate in an unrelated field.

If you are a non-traditional student, you need to realize that the basic fundamental requirements are the same. One needs to realize that all prerequisite courses need to be taken prior to taking the DAT and application. This may mean going back to school to complete those courses. This is known as post-baccalaureate studies. It is very important to do well in your post-baccalaureate courses, especially if you do not have a strong GPA for your undergraduate courses.

ഈ ഌ

Post-Baccalaureate Programs:

Post-baccalaureate or "post-bac" programs are designed for students who apply to dental school after graduating college. One can fulfill their requirements for dental school through various programs offered by many institutions.

It is very important to understand the different types of programs for your needs. Many post-bac programs cater to students wanting to enter medical school. However, one must talk to an advisor of the prospective school and discuss their motivation to go to dental school. Many students who did not complete their prerequisites during their undergrad years go back to a post-bac program to fulfill those requirements. Post-bac is ideal for those students who have graduated from an undergraduate institution, have some working experience, and now want to enter dental school. In order to enter dental school one will need to complete all of the required courses and a post-baccalaureate program will be able to fulfill those requirements. Also, this program is ideal for those individuals who did not do as well as they would have liked in undergraduate studies and now need a fresh start in showing dental schools their motivation and determination.

Before applying to any post-baccalaureate institution, the following questions need to be considered:

What is the minimum GPA needed to enter?

Is this a certificate or degree-granting program?

Can I transfer these credits to another institution or another Master's degree program?

How many of the program's students were successfully accepted to dental school?

Only enter a post-baccalaureate program if you do not have any prerequisites done. If you do have prerequisites done and just want to improve your GPA, it would be better if you complete a Master's degree in a science-related field such as Biology, Biochemistry, or a degree in Public Health.

It is also important to recognize your motivation. Going back to school again is not easy, especially if you have been out of school for a while or just did not do well. More education may be a second chance for you, but it may also be the last chance. If your GPA from undergrad is below a 3.2, then you must get above 3.5 in every class if not higher. Dental schools need to see a huge improvement in post-baccalaureate classes, as well as the DAT score to consider you a viable candidate. Remember, the students in post-baccalaureate programs are mostly trying to get into medical school and professors cater to them. In addition, some post-baccalaureate schools prep the students for the MCAT exam. Ask specific questions prior to applying and then make a decision.

Here is a complete list of programs that cater to all types of applicants:

Programs for students under-represented in the health professions:

- Associated Medical Schools of New York
- Chicago Area Health & Medical Careers Program
- Drexel University College of Medicine: Pathway to Medical School (DPMS)
- Georgetown University (GEMS)
- Michigan State University (ABLE)
- Roswell Park Graduate Division, SUNY at Buffalo
- Southern Illinois University (MEDPREP)
- The Ohio State University
- UCLA School of Medicine
- University of California Davis
- University of California Irvine
- University of California San Diego
- University of Connecticut
- University of Pittsburgh (UPIRTA)
- Wayne State
- Wake Forest University School of Medicine

Programs for students who have little or no science experience and want to take all their prerequisites after their Bachelor's degree:

    Agnes Scott College
    Bennington College
    Bryn Mawr
    Bryn Mawr (PB/MD)
    Brandeis University
    College of Liberal and Professional Students at The University of Pennsylvania
    Drexel University College of Medicine
    Duquesne University
    Georgetown University
    Goucher College
    Hofstra University
    Johns Hopkins
    La Salle University
    Long Island University
    Mills College
    Montana State University
    Mount Holyoke College
    New York University
    Northwestern University
    Pennsylvania State University
    Roosevelt College
    San Francisco State University *(Certificate Program)*
    Scripps College
    Tufts University
    University of Louisville *(Certificate Program)*
    University of Rochester
    University of Vermont
    University of Virginia
    University of Connecticut
    University of Miami
    University of Southern California

University of Maryland
Wellesley College

General Programs
Programs for students who need to improve their credentials, as well as those who have little or no science experience:

- American International College
- American University
- Assumption College
- California State University, Fullerton
- College of Liberal and Professional Students at The University of Pennsylvania
- Columbia University
- Drexel University, Medical Science Preparatory (MSP)
- Drexel University, Veterinary Medical Science (VMS)
- Duquesne University *(PBPM)*
- Harvard University Extension School
- Loyola University Chicago, Mundelein College
- Lake Erie College of Osteopathic Medicine
- New York College of Podiatric Medicine Pre-Matriculation Course
- Roosevelt College
- San Francisco State University *(Informal Post-Bac Program)*
- SUNY Stony Brook
- Temple University
- University of North Carolina at Greensboro
- University of Miami
- University of Oregon
- USC Somos Hermanos Student Immersion Program
- Virginia Commonwealth University and Medical College of Virginia
- Worcester State College

Dental Post-Baccalaureate/Master's degree programs
    Boston University
    Creighton University
    San Francisco State University
    Temple University
    University of Bridgeport
    University of California, San Francisco

Master's degree Programs
    Boston University School of Medicine
    Case Western Reserve University (MS in Anesthesia)
    Case Western Reserve University School of Medicine (BSTP)
    Columbia University (Human Nutrition)
    Dartmouth Institute for Health Policy and Clinical Practice
    Des Moines University Osteopathic and Podiatric Medicine, Health Sciences
    Drexel University College of Medicine, Master's & Post-Bac Programs (Vet too)
    Georgetown University (SMP)
    Indiana University
    Kansas City University of Medicine and Biosciences
    Loyola University Chicago, Master's in Medical Science Program
    National Institutes of Health (NIH)
    New York Institute of Technology
    New York Medical College
    New York University (NYU) (Bioethics)
    Nova Southeastern University
    Philadelphia College of Osteopathic Medicine
    Rosalind Franklin University of Medicine and Science
    Roswell Park Graduate Division, SUNY at Buffalo
    SUNY at Albany
    SUNY Upstate Medical University & Syracuse University - CNYMPH
    Syracuse University (Neuroscience)

The Commonwealth Medical College
The George Washington University, School of Public Health and Health Services
The University of Tennessee College of Graduate Health Sciences
Thomas Jefferson University
Touro University Nevada (MS in Occupational Therapy)
Tufts School of Nutrition Science & Policy (MS/PhD)
Tufts University School of Medicine (MBS)
Tufts Cumming School of Veterinary Medicine
University of Bridgeport Health Sciences
University of Buffalo, Department of Pharmaceutical Sciences
University of Buffalo, School of Medicine & Biomedical Sciences
University of California, Los Angeles *(MS or PhD in Oral Biology)*
University of Cincinnati College of Medicine (SMP)
University of Medicine and Dentistry of New Jersey
University of Wisconsin-Madison, School of Veterinary Medicine
Union Graduate College (MBA in Healthcare Management)
Union Graduate College Mount Sinai School of Medicine (Bioethics)
Wake Forest University (Bioethics)

Other Options *(Do your research)*
American Association for the Advancement of Science (AAAS)
AmeriCorps
FamiliesUSA
Mabelle Arole International Fellowship
Mayo Clinic
National Institutes of Health
NIH Undergraduate Scholarship Program
National Science Foundation (NSF)

Partners HealthCare
Peace Corps
Student Conservation Association
Teach For America

☙ ❧

CANADIAN DENTAL APPLICANTS

This section will cover some of the differences in the application process for Canadian schools. First and foremost, there are 10 Dental Schools in Canada. These are listed below.

    Laval University
    Dalhousie University
    McGill University
    University of Alberta
    University of British Columbia
    University of Manitoba
    University of Montreal
    University of Saskatchewan
    University of Toronto
    University of Western Ontario

Since there are very few dental schools in Canada, competition is higher. The average GPA is over 3.7, where the U.S. schools average is between 3.3 and 3.6. With so many people wanting to enter dental school, many apply to U.S. schools in conjunction with Canadian schools.

The prerequisites are similar to U.S. schools. One has to take the basic courses and then take the DAT. The Canadian DAT is a little different since it has an additional test called the Manual Dexterity Test, which tests on how well a candidate can use their hands. A piece of "soap" is given and the candidate has to carve certain shapes of detailed proportion. Second, the Canadian DAT does not cover Organic Chemistry or Quantitative Reasoning.

The duration of each component of the DAT is listed below:

Manual Dexterity Test .... 30 minutes

Survey of Natural Sciences Test .... 60 minutes

Perceptual Ability Test .... 60 minutes

Reading Comprehension .... 60 minutes

From the Canadian Dental Association website here is the generic scope of exams for the Canadian DAT as discussed on the Canadian Dental Association Website:

Scope of the Dental Aptitude Test

There are four examinations included in the English DAT and three examinations included in the French DAT. The tests administered include:

1. Manual Dexterity Test

Carving a specified model out of a cylindrical bar of soap specially made for the DAT.

2. Survey of Natural Sciences

Biology

Origin of life; cell metabolism (including photosynthesis); enzymology; cellular processes; thermodynamics; organelle structure and function; mitosis/meiosis; biological organization and relationship of major taxa (using the five-kingdom system: monera, planti; anamalia; protista; fungi); Vertebrate Anatomy and Physiology - structure and function of vertebrate systems (integumentary, skeletal, muscular, circulatory, immunological, digestive, respiratory, urinary, nervous/senses, endocrine, and reproductive); Developmental Biology - fertilization, descriptive embryology, and developmental mechanisms; Genetics: molecular genetics; human genetics; classical genetics; Chromosomal genetics; Evaluation, Ecology, and Behavior: natural selection; population genetics/speciation; cladistics; population and community ecology; ecosystems; animal behavior (including social).

General Chemistry

Stoichiometry and General Concepts (percent composition; empirical formulae; balancing equations; moles and molecular formulas; molecular formula weights; molar mass; density; calculations from balanced equations; gases (kinetic molecular theory of gases; Dalton's, Boyle's, Charles', and ideal gas laws); liquids and solids; (intermolecular forces; phase changes; vapor pressure; structures; polarity; properties); Solutions (polarity; properties; colligative; non-colligative; forces; concentration calculations) Acids and Bases (pH; strength; Brønsted-Lowry reactions; calculations) Chemical Equilibria (molecular; acid/base; precipitation; calculations; Le Chatelier's principle); Thermodynamics and Thermochemistry (law of thermodynamics; Hess's law; spontaneity; enthalpies and entropies; heat transfer) Chemical Kinetics (rate laws; activation energy; half-life) Oxidation-Reduction Reactions (balancing equations; determination of oxidation numbers; electrochemical calculations; electrochemical concepts and terminology) Atomic and Molecular Structure (electron configuration; orbital types; Lewis-Dot diagrams; atomic theory; quantum theory; molecular geometry; bond types; sub-atomic particles) Periodic Properties (representative elements; transition elements; periodic trends; descriptive chemistry) Nuclear Reactions (balancing equations; binding energy; decay processes; particles; terminology) Laboratory (basic techniques; equipment; error analysis; safety; data analysis).

3. Perceptual Ability

Angle discrimination, form development, cubes, orthographic projections, and apertures.

4. Reading Comprehension (English DAT only)

This part consists of three reading passages and requires the ability to read, organize, analyze, and remember new information in dental and basic sciences. Also requires the ability to comprehend thoroughly when studying scientific information. Reading materials are typical of materials encountered in the first year of dental school and require no prior knowledge of the topic other than a basic undergraduate preparation in science.

The French and English language examinations require approximately four and five hours respectively, with no formal lunch break. However, stretch breaks will be provided.

If you are a Canadian student it is advised for you to apply to AADSAS as soon as possible since it may take time for your items to be processed. Most U.S. schools will accept your Canadian DAT scores but you must be sure so there are no surprises. Some schools may require you to take the U.S. exam, but each year the criteria changes. Also, loan applications will be different so you need to find a way to finance your education if you are going to study in the U.S. Follow the same guidelines discussed in this book and you should be in good shape for the application cycle.

෩ ෪

THE INTERVIEW

The interview is a milestone in the dental admission process. Once granted, an interview shows that your "paper" application has technically been accepted. Now the admissions committee wants to see your "physical" application. The interview has many purposes and is probably the most critical assessment tool for the admissions committee. It gives the school a chance to see you for who you are, as well as the opportunity for you to see the school. Most schools put aside the GPA, the transcript, and the DAT score, and simply want to get to know you.

Here are several reasons for the interview:

See candidate's passion for dentistry
See if the candidate can communicate effectively
See if the candidate can become an asset to the field
Ask candidate ethical questions regarding certain areas of the field
Clear up any questions the committee has about the application
Answer any questions/concerns a candidate has about the program
Show the clinical environment to the candidate
Have the candidate interact with other candidates

After a thorough examination of the primary, secondary application, and the interview, the dental committee has enough information to select their incoming class. Most dental schools have selection committees who meet either after each interview date or group of dates and select the most promising candidates. A letter of admission is sent to the candidate after a certain date. For most schools the date is December 1st of the year prior to matriculation. So if you interviewed in October, the earliest you may know about your acceptance status is December 1st. Some schools may hold your acceptance until all of the possible candidates are interviewed; however this is rare.

Common Interview Questions

Below is a list of questions that may come up during the interview. These are the most common questions that interviewers ask. However, depending upon your application and life experience, they may ask different ones. Odd and off-topic questions are not uncommon. Uncomfortable questions are asked to see how you respond in stressful situations.

The basic rule of thumb is to be honest. If you do not know how to answer a question you can and should answer, "I do not know." Not everyone has the answers to every question, and that includes dentists. Do not lie or exaggerate, especially about dental experience. Honesty is always the best policy.

Sometimes negative attributes of your application are brought forward. You should not panic, but instead use this time to explain yourself. For example, if you received a low grade in a class and the interviewer asks why, you should let them know about the situation. Take responsibility for the grade, never point fingers to others, especially professors. Remember, your interviewers were college students as well and they know that everyone has certain factors which affect them in college, dental school, and beyond. The best way is to calmly explain the situation.

You should be comfortable and relaxed. Eye contact is important and being assertive by slightly nodding during the interview is appropriate. Most interviews are one-on-one; however group interviews are not uncommon. You may have two or more faculty members interviewing you, or you may have one faculty member interviewing a group of students.

Prepare yourself by jotting down some notes for the following questions. Before you go on any dental interviews, spend the night before brainstorming. Your answers must be clear and to the point. Once you have answered the question you can expand and even ask the interviewer a question. This keeps the conversation going, keeps you cool, and the interviewer engaged. Remember, preparation equals confidence. The more confidence you project, the more positive influence you shed at your interview. However, confidence should not be confused with egotistical responses. Humor is recommended but you should stay in the safe zone. Any rude or controversial topics should be avoided. If you develop good rapport with your interviewer, do not let yourself go. This is still an interview. Be amicable, but do not stray from the main reason you are there: to get accepted.

Here are some common questions which are grouped in different themes. Chances are, up to 85% of the questions will come from here. If you are prepared, you will knock the interview out of the park. Make sure you jot down ideas for each question. This way you will be able to confidently relay your thoughts.

ಸಿ ಲ

Basic questions
1) Why do you want to be a dentist?
_____
_____
_____

2) What are your hobbies?
_____
_____
_____

3) Tell me about yourself.
_____
_____
_____

4) What are your parent's professions?
_____
_____
_____

5) When did your interest in dentistry begin?

_____
_____

6) How many dental schools have you applied at?

_____
_____

7) Have you applied for other medical professions?

_____
_____

8) If you do not get into dental school this year, what is your back up plan?

_____
_____

9) Are you interested in teaching?

_____
_____

ಸಂ ಡಿ

Dental Probing Questions
Tell us about your experiences in dentistry.

_____
_____
_____

What don't you like about dentistry?
_____
_____

Is anyone in your family a dentist?
_____
_____

Where do you see yourself in five years? 10 years?
_____
_____

Do you want to specialize? If so, what area?
_____
_____

What is your favorite dental procedure?
_____
_____

Dentistry is very intensive on your hands. Do you have good manual dexterity?
_____
_____

Have you had any dental work done? What was your experience?
_____
_____
_____

In your opinion, what are the qualities of a good dentist?

___

Are you comfortable working with body fluids such as blood and saliva, while treating the oral cavity?

___

Have you had any experience handling bio-hazardous materials? If so, how did you protect yourself?

___

ಸಂ ಲ

College questions
1) Why did you major in (*enter major here*)?

___

2) What was your favorite class, as well as your least favorite class in college?

___

3) Did you go on any interesting trips in college?

___

4) What class did you do poorly in, if any?

_____
_____

5) Why did you do poorly in that subject?

_____
_____

6) How do you think you could improve your college experience?

_____
_____

7) What subjects did you or are you taking in order to prepare for dental school?

_____
_____

8) Have you failed a class?

_____
_____

9) Have you dropped out of a class?

_____
_____

☙ ❧

Volunteer and work experience

1) What volunteer experience do you have?

2) Did you shadow or work with a dentist?

3) What did you do at the dental office?

4) Did you work in college?

5) Tell us some of the jobs you had during college.

6) Have you done research? If so, where? Did you present or publish your research?

7) How do you juggle academic, social and family life?

8) How do you study?

9) Have you been involved in any leadership roles in your life?

10) What has been the most stressful situation in your life?

ఠ ఔ

Program related questions

1) Why should we select you to our program?

2) What have you heard of our program?

3) Do you know any students in this program?

4) What school is your top choice?

5) Have you spoken to any current students?

Ethical Questions

1) Suppose you were taking a test and your friend asks you for an answer. Would you tell the professor?

2) If a patient comes to you and asks you repeatedly to fill a certain prescription of a narcotic what would you say?

3) How would you describe an ethical dentist?

4) If you were drilling on a tooth and you accidentally worked on the wrong one what would you do?

5) You are trying to pull a tooth but it is too difficult or you feel you are unable to remove it. What do you do?

6) If a patient tells you he has AIDS would you still see him or her?

_____

_____

Note: For ethical questions please refer to the chapter on dental ethics. If you are asked any questions on dental ethics, answer them confidently. Always put yourself in the patient's shoes. If you were having a tooth drilled and the dentist drilled the wrong tooth what would you want? Would you want the dentist to tell you? Obviously, the answer should be yes.

So you can say: "As in all healthcare fields, mishaps happen and all dentists are human. It is not that we make mistakes, but how we take accountability for our actions. If I was in that situation and drilled the wrong tooth, I would stop and let the patient know what happened."

So use this approach in handling ethical questions. Remember, as health care professionals, people trust us to be honest and treat them how we would want to be treated.

ಐ ಡ

110 QUESTIONS ABOUT DENTAL SCHOOL

In the following pages, I have compiled a list of questions I have received through the Student Doctor Network from fellow members. These are the major questions people have about dental school and may shed light on questions regarding the aspects of the application process, specialties, and dental school in general.

1) What should I major in if I want to pursue dentistry?

This is a common question among pre-dental students. Every student who wishes to pursue healthcare thinks that majoring in a science is necessary. However, this is not always true. Dental schools love to see variety in their applicants and they really want their students to be well diverse. However, you should think about your interests. If you always wanted to learn a foreign language, undergrad is the time to do it. Do something you love. That way, you will be passionate about the subject and your interest in it will spark better grades. Remember, no matter what major you choose you must complete the prerequisites. So in turn, being a science major, especially biology, may be less work since the majority of the core requirements are covered in that major. However, you should not base your major selection based on the amount of work. Do something interesting. You don't know how many people go through undergrad and do not enjoy a single class they took. Why? Because they did not pursue their interests or listen to their heart, and therefore, their undergrad experience was spoiled. Wasting four years is not a good idea.

2.) What are the prerequisites for dental school admission?

For most dental schools the prerequisites include:
- One year of general biology
- One year of general chemistry
- One year of organic chemistry

- One year of general physics (algebra based)
- One semester of mathematics
- One semester of English/composition

However, some dental schools want their students to be ready for the advanced sciences and some require (most recommend) taking Biochemistry, Microbiology, and/or Anatomy and Physiology. It's always a good idea that students research each individual program carefully and makes sure s/he meets all prerequisite demands. If you did poorly in a class that is a prerequisite it might be a good idea to take advanced classes and do well in order to show the admission committee that you can handle the material.

3) **Do I have to complete all of my prerequisites prior to applying?**

The answer to this is no! In order to apply, you need to take the DAT. The DAT does not have physics. For this reason, one can take physics after applying and taking the DAT. However, it is in the applicant's best interest to finish all of the prerequisites as soon as possible. Also, if you want to prove to the admission committee their ability to get good grades in science classes one can do so in doing well in the prerequisite classes. Some of the higher level requirements such as Biochemistry and Microbiology may be taken after your application has been submitted. However, if advanced courses are required, you will have to provide the dental school a copy of your final transcript prior to matriculation.

4) **What is the typical application timeline for a traditional applicant?**

For a traditional student, the usual application time is between their junior and senior year, usually in the summer. If you want to matriculate right after your senior year of college you should make an aggressive effort to take their DAT, get all the recommendations, and write your personal statement as soon as possible. Obviously, this timeline will reflect when you decided to enter dentistry. Some students know they want to be dentists since they were five years old, while other students, especially non-traditional applicants may realize dentistry is for them after working for 15 years. So, each applicant is different, and dental schools try to accept students from various backgrounds.

5) Should I work at a dental clinic?

Since entry into dental school is getting more and more competitive each year, it is advisable that you have ample experience about the field. Many admission committee members look upon an applicant's experience and correlate it to their interest the field. Also, many dental schools prefer a letter of recommendation from a dental professional. Some schools even require you to turn in a log of hours that you have worked/shadowed a dentist. It would be a great idea to take notes after each opportunity to shadow a dental professional. By keeping a log, it will be easy to remember certain keywords and procedures. Also, this log system will help you recall interesting times when you are preparing for an interview.

6) Do you think dental schools like to see research?

There are many reasons why you should definitely consider doing research prior to entering dental school. By doing research, it illustrates that you have an analytical mind and can think independently and creatively. However, research is not a requirement and just like choosing a major, you should be open-minded and make sure you love the project. If you are doing research and are not interested or think it is boring, then it really does not help serve a purpose for you or the laboratory that has invited you to participate. Also, you should look at all possibilities of research. Research does not necessarily have to be science-oriented; you can focus on any aspect of research, from archaeology to neuroscience. The opportunities are endless!

7) How many hours of dental experience should I have?

It really varies. Some schools have a requirement of 50 or so hours. However, most schools do not have a set requirement. This is totally up to the applicant. Some applicants step in the dental office and fall in love, whereas other people need to explore the profession more thoroughly in order to totally grasp what the profession is all about. It is important to get ample experience because it shows that you know what you are getting yourself into and also give you more credibility at the interview.

8) **What is a good GPA/DAT scores for admission to dental school?**

About a decade ago the average DAT scores were roughly 15-16; however due to the popularity of this profession, there recently has been an increase to about 18 per section. In order to get into dental school, the averages range from 18 to 21, depending upon the school. Each school is different since they each weigh different criteria. One school may heavily look upon the PAT score, whereas another may look more toward the Science score. However, both Academic Score and PAT Score are the main determining criteria. Take a look at the GPA/DAT table in the Dental Admission Test section.

9) **Is personality or grades more important for gaining admission?**

Each school is different in this respect. Since dentistry is a well rounded profession, most dental schools select their candidates in the same way. However, it is important to realize that grades and DAT scores are the primary determining factors. Some schools have cut-offs for grades and DAT scores prior to granting you an interview. You could have the most experience in the world and have published various articles, but if your numbers do not pass the initial screening, you will most likely not be granted an interview. No interview equals no acceptance. Other schools look at all aspects of the application prior to granting you an interview. There are a few schools that do not interview their applicants, but this is very rare now in this day and age. Once you are granted an interview, it is safe to assume that your numbers are okay; however two things now determine your success:

    1. Personality
    2. Amount of spaces remaining in the class

For these reasons, applying early can increase your chances of getting in, since the class will not be full.

10) When can I take the DAT?

The DAT is administered by Thomson Prometeric (www.2test.com) in a computer format. You can take it throughout the year and various times throughout the day.

11) Whom should I contact in order to take the DAT?

When you are ready to take the DAT you can register to take the test on the internet at the ADA website (www.ada.org) or register through the mail. Applications for the DAT are usually available at the academic advising centers, pre-professional student office, dental school, or the letter of recommendation service center. However, the best way is to register is through www.ada.org. Once you register and pay the fee, you will be instructed to contact Thomson Prometric (the test administrator) and select a test date. This can be accomplished via the internet or phone.

12) Is the DAT mandatory for all schools?

Yes, the DAT is mandatory for all U.S. schools. Some U.S. schools will consider the Canadian DAT as an equal counterpart, whereas some will not. For those students who enter a combined degree program (college degree + dental degree), the DAT is usually a part of your acceptance contract, saying that when the right time comes, you must take it and sometimes score at a certain level in order to remain in the program.

13) What is the difference between the American DAT and the Canadian DAT?

The American DAT consists of six sections: Biology, Chemistry, Perceptual Ability Test, Reading Comprehension Test, and Quantitative Reasoning.

The Canadian DAT does not include Quantitative Reasoning and Organic Chemistry. However, the Canadian DAT does include Soap

Carving. Soap Carving tests the manual dexterity ability of the candidate.

14) How is the DAT scored?

Each section of the DAT is scored independently and then averaged to form the "Academic Average" score. However, the PAT score remains independent. The maximum one can get on each section is 30.

15) What are the sections of the DAT?

The American DAT consists of six sections:

    Survey of the Natural Sciences

        Biology (40 questions)

        Chemistry (30 questions)

        Organic Chemistry (30 questions)

    Perceptual Ability Test (90 questions)

    Reading Comprehension Test (50 questions)

    Quantitative Reasoning (45 questions)

16) How long do I have for each section on the DAT?

SECTION	Total amount of time allotted	Number of questions	Time to answer each question
Natural Sciences	90 min	100	0.9 min
Perceptual Ability	60 min	90	0.67 min
Reading Comprehension	60 min	50	1.2 min
Quantitative Reasoning	45 min	40	1.13 min

17) What is the most important section on the DAT?

This varies depending upon the school. Some schools weigh certain sections higher than others. However, you should try to aim for a 20 in each section.

18) **What is the importance of the PAT?**

The PAT helps the schools determine the applicant's ability to recognize and mentally manipulate shapes. This is important since dentists, unlike many other professions, work in very small spaces and must have very precise hand-eye coordination. The PAT determines how well an applicant can visually and mentally see images by testing by angle discrimination, form development cubes, orthographic projections, apertures, and paper folding. Also, radiographs are an important diagnostic tool for any dentist and it is important to turn a two dimensional image into a three dimensional image in your head.

19) **Do some schools look at one score in particular?**

Most schools mainly look at the Academic Score (overall average) and the PAT score. However, individual scores are scrutinized as well in order to determine consistent level of performance. It is always better to have 18 or above in each section than a 24 in one section and 13's in others.

20) **What if I don't do well on the DAT. Can I re-take it?**

Yes, since we have the advantage of taking the DAT at any time of the year, you can retake the DAT if you do not perform well. However, the catch is that you can only retake the DAT 90 days after your previous DAT date. That way, get a minimum of three months of study time. We have encountered many students who take the DAT with no practice or previous study-time, in terms to get a "feel" for the exam. However, this is not advisable. It is better to prepare and take the exam when you feel confident enough to succeed. This test can be very grueling, and it is much better to slay it in one time rather than two or three!

21) **If I retake the DAT, does the admission committee look down upon that?**

If you retake the DAT one thing is for sure: you must improve! Most admission committees will compare both scores and want to see improvement on your most recent attempt. If you must retake the DAT, it is a good idea to contact admission directors and ask them directly for consultation of your projective goal on your next exam. Most admission directors would be happy to discuss your scores and applications, and will tell you directly what you should hit the second time around for serious consideration (hint: usually admissions directors will tell you to hit 20's across).

22) Where do I take the DAT?

The DAT is administered at various Thompson Prometric Sites (www.2test.com) which are located throughout the U.S. Usually, most of them are combined with Sylvan Learning Centers.

23) When is the DAT offered?

The DAT is offered year round! If you are interested in taking the DAT, once you have registered it is your responsibility to set up an appointment to take it. You can schedule the exam in the morning or afternoon on any day you want (as long the testing center has availability)!

24) Can I choose to take the DAT on paper or computer?

Since 1998, the DAT has been exclusively administered on the computer. However, if you have a "special accommodation" request, then you must contact the testing service and ask them in writing if you want to take the test on paper. This option is now rare and the testing centers will accommodate students with disabilities.

25) When do I get my scores?

Another convenient thing about the DAT testing experience is that you get the scores immediately upon completing the test battery. The testing proctor will emboss the scores to make them official.

26) What will my scores look like?

Unfortunately, the scores are not very detailed. They just state your individual score for each section, plus an academic score and a science score. If you have questions about your scores or want to have them re-graded by hand, then you must contact the ADA in writing within 30 days of your test.

27) How long before schools receive my scores?

Usually it takes the schools two to three weeks to receive the scores. However, just because you got your scores does not mean the schools have them, as it might take them several days or weeks to sort out the mail. Some schools mail systems are very slow, so also take that into account.

28) How many credits/units should I have prior to applying to a dental school?

Usually 90 semester credits or 135 quarter credits are needed prior to applying to dental school.

29) Can I apply after three years of undergraduate schooling?

Yes, most schools will consider applicants right out of junior year of college. However, it is more competitive to gain admission since most (over 90%) of applicants will have a Bachelor's degree upon entering dental school. Therefore, it is crucial for these applicants to have stellar numbers.

30) How competitive is getting into Dental School?

There are about 4,100 seats in all of the U.S. dental schools. Usually around 10,000 – 15,000 applications are submitted each year. However, due to the increasing popularity of dentistry, the competition is increasing each year. Even though the quantity of applicants remains quite stable, the quality of applicants is increasing. For this reason, it is to the applicants' advantage to apply early, get good grades, and do well on the DAT.

31) What is the male to female ratio in dental school?

Dentistry was once a male dominated profession. Nowadays, dentistry is an attractive field for women. The ratio of men to women in the field is almost even at 50:50. There are slightly more males working; however, that may change soon.

32) What is AADSAS?

AADSAS is a part of the American Dental Education Association (www.adea.org). AADSAS stands for Associated American Dental

Schools Application Service and is a standardized application for all American Dental Schools and some Canadian dental schools. Usually the dental application is available between mid-May and early March of the following year. AADSAS takes your application, transcripts, and letters of recommendations and forwards them to the schools of your choosing. This service batches all of the components of each applicant together to give the dental school a "bird's eye" view of the application. In turn, it is more efficient for the schools to screen the applicants.

33) Can I apply to schools without applying through AADSAS?

Other than the Texas dental schools and a few others, all other American dental schools require AADSAS for your application submission. However, if you wish to apply to Canadian schools there are some that you can apply directly.

34) What is the typical application time period?

Usually, the typical time period is between June of the year prior to matriculation and March of the year of matriculation. However, each school is different. Some schools have deadlines in November or December of the year prior to matriculation. So for this reason, you should carefully plan in advance when to send all the required materials.

35) How many schools should I apply to?

This is a very tough question, since it really varies. There are various factors you must consider, especially your grades and DAT scores. If you are an average applicant, you should apply between five to 10 schools. However, if you are a below average applicant, you may want to diversify, research your schools, and apply to more than 10. You should also consider where you would like to practice and where you would want to go to school. Applying to schools for the sake of getting in should not be a priority. Since dental school is a huge investment of time and money, you should select your school very carefully so that you will be content in that environment.

36) How many dental schools are there in the U.S. and Canada?

There are 58 accredited dental schools in the U.S. and 10 in Canada. There are several more opening up in a few years.

37) How can I improve my chances?

There are several ways to improve your chances for acceptance. The best way is to apply early and be organized. We can't tell you how many great applicants wait until the last minute to apply and do not get in anywhere. Also, getting good recommendations is always a great way to increase your chances. For this, you'll need to interact with professors and do well in their classes.

38) Is applying earlier better?

Yes, for the average applicant applying early will always give you the benefit. Even if you haven't taken your DAT or gotten all your recommendations, applying as soon as you can is a very important. Remember, it generally takes four to six weeks for your application to be processed by AADSAS and submitted to the schools. So if you strategically plan it out, then you could apply and take the DAT within a month of submitting the application and still have all your scores and numbers ready to be evaluated.

39) How important is the admissions essay?

By the time you apply, your GPA and DAT scores are set in stone. The admission essay is an invaluable tool which lets you discuss other parts of your application. The essay should be taken very, very seriously. Basically, here you have a canvas and you can paint any type of picture you want for the admission committee.

40) What should I talk about in the admission's essay?

You can illustrate your potential to be a compassionate dentist, or you could illustrate extenuating circumstances that make you unique and an asset to the field. Also, the admission essay can also be used to explain certain downfalls you might have had, which impacted your grades. You are in control.

41) What is an application fee?

The dental school application process is not only time consuming, but also very expensive. Many people think that once they applied through AADSAS they have paid their fees. However, to their dismay, they do not hear from any schools or get postcards illustrating that their file is incomplete since they have not submitted their application fees. After the schools receive your AADSAS application some will send you a supplementary application/secondary application. This is an application which is unique to the school itself. Along with the application, you must send the application fee. This fee ranges between $25 to around a $100. Also, it is advised to verify which schools want the fee submitted immediately and to whom the check should be made out to. If you are organized and manage your time wisely this should not be a problem.

42) What are secondary applications?

Secondary applications are unique to the individual school and usually are sent out for two reasons:

    a) The AADSAS application has been received, or
    b) The applicant has passed an initial screening.

Most schools only give secondary applications to applicants whom they are serious about. It is up to the applicant to submit the secondary application and associated fees immediately. Some schools even stamp the date on the secondary application that it was sent out and stamp it again to see when they receive it. That way, they can analyze how serious an applicant is in their program (the faster they receive it shows interest and determination).

43) Can I get secondary applications prior to applying to AADSAS?

No, most schools will only mail out secondary applications after receiving your AADSAS application. However, there are some schools that have their secondary applications on their website. These schools usually screen the applications using the secondary applications.

44) What if I don't get a secondary?

There could be several reasons why you might not receive a secondary application. There are many schools that do not have secondary applications, but solely rely on the AADSAS application. However, don't be confused since these schools also require application fees which usually are sent at the same time you submit your AADSAS application. The main one might be that your file is incomplete (missing transcripts, letters of recommendation, or application fees). However, if your file is complete and you do not receive a secondary, there might be a chance that you did not make the preliminary screening. This issue is best resolved by directly contacting the school and discussing your concern with the admissions director.

45) What is an interview?

After your file is complete, the school will review it and deem if you deserve an interview. An interview is a very honorable achievement because it shows that the school is very serious about you. It is advisable to interview as soon as possible. Some schools will not let you choose a date and they give you an interview date.

46) Are there schools that don't interview?

Yes, there are a few schools that do not have formal interviews, but they strongly suggest you visit the school prior to making your final decision. However, there are several schools that have regional interviews throughout the United States.

47) Do schools pay for travel expenses?

No, schools do not pay for travel expenses. However, they may pay for lunch!

48) What should I wear to an interview?

Since interviews are a formal affair, you should dress elegantly and professionally. Men should wear suits and neck ties. Women should dress in a professional fashion.

49) How long should I stay?

Even though the interview itself usually is less than one hour long, the school invites the applicant for the entire day to tour the facilities, discuss financial matters, and talk with current students. However, if possible, you should stay an extra day or two to absorb the environment and get more feedback from the current students.

50) What should I look for in a school during the interview?

There are various things one should look for during the interview. First and foremost, you should see if the school's environment is comfortable for you. Ask the current students how their experience is going. Ask about the pros and cons. There is no reason why you should not stay and investigate the school, the staff and the students.

51) When is the first day I will find out if I get accepted?

Dental schools have an agreement that they will not tell students before a certain day that they have been accepted. They do this out of consideration for both the schools and applicant. They want the applicant to attend the interviews and to see the programs, and get a feel for each schools uniqueness and personality. Many students may miss out if they are told of an early admission and cancel the rest of their interviews. Typically students find out whether they have been accepted on December 1st. Often times, schools will send out letters so that they reach the applicant on December 1st or even call first thing in the morning to tell the applicant that they were accepted.

52) If I get an acceptance letter, what is the next step?

If you receive an acceptance letter, the first thing you should do is celebrate! Getting accepted is an awesome feeling and accomplishment. Once you have celebrated, read through all the material. Admissions offices include what the next step is for students. If you were accepted in December, chances are you have 45 days to make a decision. There are forms which you will have to fill out and a deposit that will have to be sent to hold a seat for you. If you were accepted later than December, the amount of time you have to decide is less, but the admissions committee will inform you how long you have to decide. Many students who interviewed at several schools during the fall receive multiple acceptances and then decide which school they are going to attend once the acceptances come in the mail. Taking your time can help you decide what the right school for you is.

53) Can I accept multiple school offers?

In a nutshell the answer is yes. However, this is greatly frowned upon. In the end, you can only attend one school, and by accepting multiple offers you are not only spending a lot of money on deposits, but you are also taking up seats that other deserving students could use. You can't be enrolled in two different dental schools at the same time, so why accept multiple offers? If you do make a deposit and then realize that another school is a better fit for you, then making the switch is acceptable. But if you are just securing a seat because it was offered, you're really hurting other students.

54) What do I do if I get accepted to a school, while I'm still waiting for my top choice to respond?

Although it's great to be accepted, if you don't get into your top choice, would you be happy at one of the other schools you applied to? The best thing to do is to evaluate your position. What's your second choice? If you haven't heard from your top choice, you can always call and ask what the status of your application is. Sometimes mail takes time. Ask the admissions office if the admissions committee has made a decision or when they are going to review your application. Give the school some time before you immediately place a deposit with another school. You and your wallet will be glad you waited.

55) Do my grades matter after I get accepted to a dental school?

Once you are accepted, your grades do matter. In fact, if you read your acceptance letter closely, there will a line saying that the acceptance is contingent upon the satisfactory completion of all courses. Although the school knows that once applicants are accepted there may be a drop in the GPA, they do expect that you will continue to perform at a decent level. Admissions committees have revoked acceptances because of failure and poor performance after acceptance. So hang in there.

56) Do I need to finish my degree after my acceptance?

Many students tend to receive a Bachelor's degree before matriculating into dental school. Some obtain a Masters degree or even a PhD before starting dental school. As far as completing your degree, so long as you complete all the required courses for dental school and have completed at least 90 semester hours or the equivalent (this is the minimum at most schools), you will be considered for admission. If you receive admission before completing your degree, you can attend so long as you meet all the requirements. Keep in mind that you are close to finishing the degree, and seeing a diploma on the wall will remind you that you reached another milestone. Always, let the dental school know you may not complete the degree and if that is okay.

57) I wrote that I will have two degrees next year. Once I've been accepted, can I drop one degree?

Yes, you can. So long you will have completed all the required courses for admission, you should have no problem dropping one of the degrees and attending dental school. However, call the school you have been accepted to and ask what they advise. As long as the school doesn't have a problem and you complete all the requirements for the dental program, you should be alright.

58) What should I do prior to dental school?

The one piece of advice I got from many students in dental school was to relax as much as possible before starting dental school. Once you are in the program, you will be extremely busy. Do some of the things you've always wanted to do before starting dental school. Travel and hang out with friends. If you want, you can even get a job. Although most people suggest just taking it easy, it really depends on what you want to do. Just make sure you stay on top of all the things that require your attention for matriculation, such as getting a physical, securing housing, and any miscellaneous paper work.

59) What classes are recommended but not required for most dental schools?

This is a very common question. Every school is different. While many schools have the same general requirements, many schools have various recommended classes. Most schools will suggest taking additional science classes such as Immunology, Anatomy, Physiology, Microbiology, Genetics, and Virology. Other schools will recommend taking more sociology classes, business classes, human diversity, and foreign language classes. In addition, dental schools are starting to recommend General Psychology and Developmental Psychology courses.

60) How important is manual dexterity?

As many people will tell you, dentistry is the marriage of science, art, and compassion for people. Manual dexterity is one of the most critical parts of this equation. In order to perform any type of dental procedure, you will need to work with your hands, mirrors, and fine instruments. If you are not capable of working with your hands or manipulating objects with a mirror, practice will help. But without the manual dexterity, you cannot perform competent dentistry. No matter how comforting and knowledgeable you may be, if you cannot perform the procedure the patient won't have any use for your expertise.

61) What can I do to improve my manual dexterity?

Practice. The key to improving your manual dexterity is by getting used to working with the instruments and seeing how they work under different circumstances. While preparing for the DAT many people play with Lego's, build model cars, or paint pictures to improve their hand-eye coordination.

62) What if I have big hands; can I be a successful dentist?

Pudgy hands, big hands, or small hands – you can't trade them in for new ones. Personally, I have seen many skilled surgeons with stubby little hands, and many with long, thin hands. You can be very successful as long as you work at it. You don't need to fit your fist into the patient's mouth, so long as you are in control and are confident your hands. Like practicing manual dexterity, the only way you will get better with your hands is by using them. Many people wonder if they will be able to type on a keyboard with big hands. In the age of laptops and small electronic devices, people have adjusted to compensate and learn to make do with what they have.

63) What is the difference between a D.M.D. and D.D.S degree?

Many people, including dentists, are confused over the use of the D.D.S. and D.M.D. degrees. Today, some dental schools grant a D.D.S. degree while others prefer to award the D.M.D. degree instead. The training the dentists receive is very similar but the degree granted is different.

Ancient medicine was divided into two groups: 1) the surgery group that dealt with treating diseases and injuries using instruments; and 2) the medicine group that dealt with healing diseases using internal remedies. Originally there was only the D.D.S. degree which stands for Doctor of Dental Surgery.

This all changed in 1867 when Harvard University added a dental school. Harvard University only granted degrees in Latin. Harvard did not adopt the D.D.S. or Doctor of Dental Surgery degree because the Latin translation was Chirurgae Dentium Doctoris or C.D.D. The people at Harvard thought that C.D.D. was cumbersome, so a Latin scholar was consulted. The scholar suggested the ancient Medicinae Doctor be prefixed with Dentariae. This is how the D.M.D. or "Dentariae Medicinae Doctor" degree was started. (Congratulations! Now you probably know more Latin than most dentists!)

At the turn of the century, there were 57 dental schools in the U.S. but only Harvard and Oregon awarded the D.M.D. In 1989, 23 of the 66 North American dental schools awarded the D.M.D.

The American Dental Association is aware of the public confusion surrounding these degrees and has tried on several occasions to reduce this confusion. Several sample proposals include: 1) eliminate the D.M.D. degree; 2) eliminate the D.D.S. degree; or 3) eliminate both degrees and invent a brand new degree that every dental school will agree to use. Unfortunately, this confusion may be with us for a long time. When emotional factors like school pride and tradition arise, it is difficult to find a compromise.

64) How long will it take me to complete dental school?

In the U.S, most dental schools are four years long. This is if you are just asking about dental school, and not thinking of residency or specialization. Dental school is very challenging, as you are not only learning medical curriculum, but you are also in the simulation laboratory learning how to perform procedures. In essence, many dentists relate their dental school experience to that of medical school but with residency being done during those four years.

65) What can I expect the first and second year of dental school?

Although the curriculum various from school to school, the first two years of dental school are spent learning the basic sciences and procedures.

66) What can I expect the third and fourth years of dental school?

In most schools, this is where your exposure to clinical dentistry begins. Although many schools have started getting students into the clinics early, the main focus of the third and fourth year are to expose students to the vast cases they will see when they begin to practice dentistry. This is also the time when students will get to interact with real patients and perform procedures on them. During the last two years of dental school there will be classes that are geared towards what you are doing in the clinic. Also, many schools have a requirement of how many procedures must be performed before you can graduate and sit for the licensing exam.

67) Does one have to do residency after dental school?

No. If you are interested in becoming a general dentist, you do not have to do a residency after dental school. However, doing a residency is becoming more popular even if you are considering becoming a general practitioner of dentistry. Further training will only strengthen your knowledge and make you that much more confident in you procedures and skill. States like New York are requiring one year of GPR (General Practice Residency) in order to practice. Some states are letting people practice with one year residency in lieu of even passing the licensing boards.

68) What different specialties are there in dentistry?

There are several specialties within the medical specialty of dentistry. There is pedodontics which is the specialty of pediatric dentistry or dentistry for children. There is orthodontics, which involves the moving and spacing of the teeth over time to create an environment for ideal dentition. There is periodontics, which is the specialty of dentistry relating to the gingival (gums) and protecting them from disease and decay, which saves the teeth. There is endodontics, the specialty which involves saving teeth that are on the verge of death, and thus removing the nerve and infection. Another specialty is Oral and Maxillofacial Facial Surgery, which involves facial reconstruction and working with severe trauma to removing impacted wisdom teeth. There is prosthodontics which is advanced prosthetics including orbital prosthesis for cancer patients. Also, there are lesser known ones such as oral pathology and oral radiology. Any dental curriculum will expose you to all of these specialties and if you find one fascinating, you may want to pursue more advanced knowledge after dental school.

69) Can a general dentist perform the same procedures as a specialist?

Although a general dentist can perform the same procedures as a specialist, often times the general dentist will do the less severe cases. Specialists have dedicated their life to becoming experts in one particular field of dentistry and have taken additional efforts to learn more about that field in the form of a residency.

70) Can a specialist perform procedures of a general dentist?

There are some specialists who continue doing certain procedures they feel comfortable with, even if they are considered outside their specialty. It is not unusual to see a periodontist extract teeth or a prosthodontist do fillings. However, in most cases specialists abide by their specialty and focus solely on what they trained to do.

71) What do I need to do if I am interested in specializing?

If you are already thinking about specializing, then you should be aware that you first need to get into and through dental school. In addition, you need to be near the top of your class in dental and perform well on the NDBE Part I and II. The best thing you can do if you are interested in specializing is learn about the specialty, and then research the schools which offer post-doctorate programs in that specialty. There are several schools which offer programs for various specialties, and although all will prepare you for the specialty, some may give you more exposure and opportunity than other programs. Another great way to learn about specializing is by calling a few of the prospective programs, let them know you have an interest in pursuing a specialization after dental school, and ask if there is anyone who you can guide you. This often helps establish a rapport, connection, and shows the school/program you are doing everything from your end to gain admission to a post-doctorate specialty program.

72) Can anyone specialize?

Once you have completed dental school, you can specialize. Specializing is competitive, and takes additional years of schooling. As long as you were in the top third of your dental class and passed the NDBE I and II with high marks, obtaining admission to a specialty should be within reach. When it comes time to specialize, you will once again be applying to programs and going on interviews. The most important part of securing a seat in a specialty program is to have great letters of recommendation, a great dental school GPA, and good NDBE I and II scores.

73) How long is specialty training?

The duration of a specialty all depends on the specialty you are interested in pursuing. There are some specialty programs that are two to three years, such as orthodontics, endodontics, and periodontics. Other specialties like oral surgery can take from four to seven years depending on the program and school you attend for specialization. There are also combined specialties like prosthodontic-periodontics that have five-year residencies.

74) What are the main criteria post-graduate programs look for?

Just like applying to dental school, post-doctorate programs are looking for qualified applicants that demonstrate they have a great interest in dentistry, particularly in a specific field of dentistry. The admissions committee for post-doctorate programs will want to see an applicant who performed well in dental school, on the NDBE part I and II, who has excellent letters of recommendation (especially from faculty in the specialty they are seeking admission), and show that they were actively involved in dental school. It would be to your advantage to gain exposure in the form of an externship during one of your breaks in dental school, or even conducting research in that field with faculty while in dental school.

75) What is the most competitive specialty?

Getting through dental school is a feat in and of itself. Currently, the most competitive residency programs are orthodontics or pedodontics. Gaining admission to all residencies are competitive; the top two or three students generally get placement in orthodontic residency, while those in the top 10 can obtain residencies in Oral Maxillofacial Surgery.

76) Does the reputation of the school influence success in finding a specialty spot?

There have been extensive debates as to whether attending a "big name school" hinders or helps obtain a position in a post-doctorate residency program. The truth is, regardless of which dental school you attend, you will have to do well. You will have to perform at the top of your class and score well on the NDBE, which are standardized tests. Just like applying to dental schools and the DAT was the evening factor, the NDBE is an evening factor for all those who are applying for residency programs. Schools with great names oftentimes have a great name because they help their students, whether it is through exposure or guiding them. They have earned a reputation and oftentimes it comes down to the way the students perform on the NDBE part I and II, as well as how many students are admitted to post-doctorate specialty programs.

77) How important is research in dental school?

This is another question pre-dental students often ask. The answer applies equally to both pre-dental and dental student: if you do not like doing research don't do it. Research is meant to give you exposure and insight on specific topics, and can be impressive on your résumé. Many of the competitive programs like to see research experience, but if you have other things to offer besides research, they will take that into account. Otherwise, it's an opportunity to learn more, but not the most critical part of dental school.

78) How are most dental schools organized?

Most dental schools have a four-year long program which awards either a D.M.D. or D.D.S. The first two years of the dental program are mainly spent learning the basic sciences and introducing the students to various aspects of dentistry, such as dental anatomy, along with laboratory skills (depending on school, you may start having clinical experience your first day, or none until third year). The last two years of dental school are predominantly spent in the clinics, seeing patients and doing procedures. Although there is a requirement at many schools, at some schools the philosophy is as soon as you understand the theory of a procedure and can perform it competently, you pass that procedure. For exam at some schools, a student must complete 10 endodontic procedures to graduate. At another dental school a student must complete endodontic procedures until the faculty is convinced the student is competent. This could mean the student does two endodontic cases or 30 endodontic cases. Also, most dental schools have post-doctorate specialty programs that train dental graduates (D.M.D./D.D.S.) to become specialists. Many dental schools also have students who pursue a doctorate but have an interest in research and allow/guide them to pursue a Ph.D. Of course, each dental school is different. Some schools have the dental and medical students take all or some basic science courses together, while at other dental schools students are given full attention and do not have to compete for faculty attention. Furthermore, most universities with a dental school share instructors/faculty members between the medical, veterinary, and health professional school students.

79)   What is the grading like in dental school?

Just like in high school and during your undergraduate education, you will have tests and receive grades in dental school. Many schools have exams on a regular basis, and grade using the alphabet system (A, B, C, D, and E/F). Other schools will have a Pass/Fail grading system. Recently, there has been an addition to some of the schools that have the Pass/Fail, which includes Honors. Now some of these schools have Honors/Pass/Fail. As far as grading is concerned on exams, most of the exams are multiple choice, so partial credit is out. Also, grading is subjective. At some dental schools an 80% is a C, while at others it is a solid B. It all depends. It also depends on the class and the professor.

80) What is the difference between research-oriented and clinical-oriented dental schools?

This is a big difference and could very well be the reason you attend or do not attend a particular school. While many dental schools believe that a dental education should include vast amounts of exposure to dentistry, they often focus on how the information will be instructed to their students. A research- oriented school is more interested in training the future dental faculty and professors. While these dental students do learn clinical procedure, the emphasis is placed on doing dental research and exploring new things. These schools want their students to be in the lab conducting experiments, writing papers and getting published. On the other hand clinically oriented school is focused on training their students to be efficient and effective practitioners of dental medicine. These schools often have students performing several procedures and are very particular about the work each student does. While there are these two extremes, it is also important to note many schools are in between. Many schools believe that the only way for a practitioner of dental medicine to be completely trained is for them to be exposed to both, and allow the student to make the decision on which path they will choose. In essence, picking a school and its program solely depends on what interests you. Some schools receive large grants from the government to conduct research; so many faculty members are engrossed in research activities as well as teaching.

81) Are there some schools that are Pass/Fail?

Yes! There are several schools that offer Pass/Fail grading systems. Whether this is good or not depends on your own preference. Some people believe that a Pass/Fail system makes the students lazy and doesn't make them work to their fullest potential. Others believe that this system takes away the innate competitiveness of a class (which can be good or bad depending on how you feel about competition) and puts the focus on just learning the material. For those who feel that Pass/Fail doesn't distinguish the class very much, Honors was introduced. So now at some schools, the grading is Honors/Pass/Fail. Many critics believe this is essentially a pushback to the original A, B, C, D and E/F grading system.

82) How many credits/units can I expect to take in dental school?

You are about to enter a doctorate program. That being said, you should expect to be inundated with a plethora of information and courses. Pursuing a doctorate is not for the faint-hearted. On average, you will take 54 credits per year.

83) What if I don't feel comfortable with procedures right out of dental school?

Although many students who graduate do feel somewhat apprehensive about practicing on private patients in the real world, it does not mean you are not prepared. Dental school is designed to give you all the knowledge and skills to be a competent and attentive practitioner of dental medicine. However, if you do feel that you need further training or that you want to more exposure there are post-doctorate programs. Many students apply for either a GPR or AEGD. A GPR is a General Practice Residency and an AEGD is Advanced Education in General Dentistry. Both have been designed to give students the opportunity to perform further clinical dentistry and learn to handle more complex cases. Another option is to go into private practice with an older dentist who will act as a mentor and help you become more comfortable with the procedures. It is normal to question your ability, but after completing dental school and passing the boards you are ready to practice dentistry.

84) What is the NDBE?

The NDBE stands for National Dental Board Exam. These are standardized board exams that every dental student takes. There are two parts: the first one given after the second year of dental school, and the second part at the end of the fourth year. It is required for every student in the U.S. to sit for the NDBE to practice and to pass dental school.

85) What is the difference between NDBE Part I and NDBE Part II?

Once again, in order to practice you must take both parts of the National Dental Board Exam. Part I is offered after completion of your basic science curriculum, and is often taken after the second year of dental school. Part I is all on the basic sciences. Part II is taken towards the end of the fourth year of dental school right before graduation. Part II covers all the clinical aspects of dentistry, including performing and explaining certain procedures.

86) What are the requirements to take the NDBE Parts I and Parts II?

The biggest requirement is completing the required courses, similarly to the DAT. Some schools will not allow you to take the NBDE until you have successfully passed the required courses.

87) When are NDBE Parts I and Parts II offered?

The NBDE is offered similarly to the DAT on the computer on almost any day of the year. You will have to register through www.ada.org and then schedule to take the exam through Thomson Prometric centers.

88) Can I repeat them if I do not pass or unhappy with my scores?

Yes. In fact, if you do not pass, you must retake them. At many schools you will not be allowed to continue without passing the NDBE. Even if you partially fail the NDBE, you must retake that part before continuing with dental school.

89) If I pass both NDBE Part I and Part II can I practice dentistry?

Not immediately, but eventually. When you graduate you get a D.M.D./D.D.S., but it's useless until you get a license from a state to practice. The state licensing boards grant licenses to those who pass the exam they determine. Some states like Florida have their own state exams. A few states are taking multiple exams like Massachusetts. Massachusetts takes all the regional clinical exams CRDTS/NERB/SRTA/WREB. Things are slowly changing every year.

90) What are regional boards?

In order to be licensed and practice in a particular state, you need to take the regional or state board exam. Once completing dental school, you must sit for the board exam to practice. Although there are regional boards that allow you to practice in several states, there are some states that do not accept regional board exams and require a special board exam to practice in that state (Florida, for example).

91) Does each state also have an independent exam?

No. Some states such as Florida have their own independent exams. Most states accept a regional board, which licenses a dentist to practice in a group of states. For instance, if you go to dental school in the Northeast U.S., you will sit for the Northeast Regional Board (NERB). The NERBs will allow you to practice in a variety of states including NY, PA, CT, NJ, DC, etc.

92) What is the difference between GPR and AEGD?

Oftentimes, people will go through dental school and not hear about the GPR/AEGD until the very end. A GPR is a General Practice Residency. An AEGD is an Advanced Education in General Dentistry. Both of these programs are geared towards those who are interested in practicing general dentistry. Basically, it is one year of advanced training after dental school where you may work in a hospital setting and rotate through different areas.

93) How long is a GPR, and what I expect to gain from it?

First of all, you should do well in dental school in order to get your choice of GPRs. There are a lot of them out there, and some are better than others. You'll end up being the ultimate chooser of which one is best for you based on a combination of what they're offering and what your looking for (i.e. some may have more oral surgery than others, some may have more O.R. time than others, some may have more intense call schedules than others). The best way to get a feel for what the program is like is to talk to the current residents sometime between January and June. As for the long term benefits of a GPR vs. going straight out into private practice, a GPR will expose you to a lot more extreme things than you'll see in private practice, which makes private practice then seem more routine day to day. A GPR will allow you improve your speed and start to learn how to manage your schedule better. A GPR will likely also expose you to different schools of thought about techniques for different procedures than you learned in dental school. However, a private practice situation where you have a strong mentor can also give this.

94) After graduation how and when do I start working?

This is a tough question and each case is different for every dentist. Some dental graduates have family members with whom they can work with. Other dentists look for jobs in the newspaper. Regardless, there is a steep need for dentists throughout the U.S. and there is no shortage of jobs. However, if you are picky and want to work in a very popular area, it may be difficult to find a job. However, if you plan ahead and talk to alumni and dentists in the area you are interested in you are sure to find a job.

95) What if I don't want to practice clinical dentistry. Are there other fields in dentistry open for me?

Surprisingly enough, many dentists come out of dental school, or even are in practice and decide they don't want to practice clinical dentistry. Does this mean they don't belong in the dental profession? Absolutely not! There are several dentists who feel that clinical practice isn't for them. As a dentist you can go back to the university and teach, do research, consult, work at a pharmaceutical company or a dental company, manage other dental offices, or even work for a non-profit organization. The possibilities are endless, but these are just a few options.

96) If I have a dental degree from a country outside the United States, how can I practice dentistry in the U.S.?

Unlike many other professions where taking a licensing exam and board exams certify you to practice, dentistry requires all foreign-trained dentists to not only pass the NDBE part I and II but also take a two or three- year course specifically for foreign-trained dentists. Since many dentists have been in practice for some time and don't remember everything from dental school, it often takes time to prepare for the NDBE part I (generally a year or so). Just like dental school, these programs are competitive, and require the dentist to take the NDBE part I and II, TOEFL, submit an application and fee, submit references if required, and supply a copy of your diploma and academic transcript. You may need to translate their transcript by an agency.

97) What schools offer advanced standing programs?

There are several schools that offer advanced standing program for foreign-trained dentists. Not all of them are the same length – some are two years, others three. New York University offers a three-year advanced standing program.

98) Can I simultaneously apply to both medical and dental school?

This is a double-edged sword. If you aren't sure what you want to do applying to both medical and dental school will just make matters worse. First off, both are enormous commitments financially and time wise. Another thing, you will be taking the seat of a person who has already devoted themselves to the service of medicine or dentistry if you do gain admission. The answer to whether you can apply to medical and dental school at the same time is: yes. However, both medical schools and dental school strongly discourage applicants from doing so, and dislike when they see an applicant who is applying to both. Even if you have a genuine interest in both, take a year off and then apply once you have made a decision. In regards to applying to both programs, when you are filling out the primary application there will be a question if you are applying to medical or dental school. If you are applying to both and lie that you aren't, the schools can still check and some schools make it a point to ask you at the interview.

99) How should I choose a school?

Oftentimes, applicants apply to several schools to guarantee that they at least get admitted to one program. Many, much to their surprise, get into more than they ever expected, and are then faced with what never appeared to be a problem: deciding which school to attend. When deciding on which school to choose you need to consider everything. What school offered the type of program that most interested you? How were you treated? How were the students treated? Were many of the students happy? How were the facilities and the faculty? Did you like the location? How much will it cost? Will you need loans? Do you have family/friends close by for support? Will you need any special requirements? Choosing a school is very personal and the reasons people attend certain schools vary from the prestige or name of a school to the student body to the clinical set up. Keep everything in perspective; the most important thing should be those things that matter to you.

100) Do dental schools have a problem if you previously applied to medical or dental school?

If you are a re-applicant to professional school, even if you are re-applying to the same professional program, or if you made the switch from one program to another, as long as you explain what made you change, show that you have thought things out thoroughly, and are certain of your choice, the schools will not hold that against you. People learn things about themselves and about life and make changes all the time. The admissions committees understand that people are people, and students are people as well.

If you decided to apply to dental school and were a previous medical school applicant do not pretend you were not. Also, prove to the committee you are committed with hours of dental volunteer experience. A letter of recommendation from a dentist who can talk about your enthusiasm for dentistry or skill will help immensely. If you are a dental school re-applicant, as long as you have improved your application with either better DAT scores, GPA, letter of recommendation, or volunteering you should also have nothing to worry about. You can tell them that you applied before and that you are determined to become a dentist. Schools like to see a motivated applicant, someone with determination. If you were in either of these positions, don't shy away from your past, just make sure you can explain it well and the school can see your passion.

101) How long should I spend at a school while interviewing?

Many students make the mistake of flying in for the interview and then flying out the same day. The reason many times is to save a few bucks on lodging or perhaps to get back to school, work, or home. If you are investing the time, money, and effort to interview at a school spend a day or few days looking at the school after your interview. If you can arrive early and get a feel for the city/town and the university, the entire trip will be much more vivid when you have to make a decision. Many schools interview on a Friday or Monday, thus giving the student the chance to spend the weekend or come a day early and get a feel for the school. If possible, we recommend spending at least an extra day. Talk with students, look around on your own, and take in the surroundings. A lot of students who spend the extra time find it to well worth the extra money and truly gives them more information. Consider the fact that you are investing the next four years of your life, not to mention your education (the biggest investment you can make). And remember, the more you learn about the school in general, the better your choice will be. Many students in retrospect wish they had done this because they didn't realize that much of what they learned on their interview wasn't the entire story. Also remember to take notes after you get out of your interview. Making a pros and cons sheet after each interview will help you rank your schools and refresh your memory once those acceptance letters start rolling in. Give yourself the extra day or so. Then you will be certain which school is right for you when you have to make decision.

102) How intense is dental school?

This is a very common question. Dental school is very intense. In addition to learning a heavy science curriculum, dental students have to practice techniques that are needed for clinical application. Many students begin their day around 8am, and often finish around 5pm. On top of this, you often spend several hours studying. Intensity of the program varies from student to student and school to school. Those who have a science background and a curriculum that eases students through the sciences will feel that dental school is very balanced. Students who had very little exposure than the required science classes and are attending schools with a curriculum that stresses sciences will feel burdened and continually under the gun.

103) How committed are the dental schools to my success?

This question is brought up by many nervous students. Your success is not just your concern but also the schools'. Unfortunately, not all schools are as ambitious for you as you would hope. The best thing for you to do is to ask an admissions director or read the schools policy on helping students. Another key indication may be the attrition rate. Oftentimes, schools with high attrition rate put a lot of blame on students. Although there are some students who do slack off, there are programs that aren't right for certain students. It is best to ask about the attrition rate, why it is what it is, what steps the school takes in helping students, and what the school does to help student who are having academic difficulty. It is your responsibility to find out where you will stand as a student. Some schools will give you a lot of help, while others will show you to the door.

104) If a student makes a commitment to the program, what is the responsibility of the faculty?

Many schools believe that doctorate students should be treated like adults, and give them due respect. This includes treating the student like a doctor in training, and working to foster a close knit relationship between the faculty and students. Although programs are changing, some schools believe the faculty is there to present the information and proctor the exams. Perhaps some faculty will assist you. As grim as this may sound, these types of schools are in the minority. Many leading programs are emphasizing that faculty should have an instructive and effective role, as opposed to an inspective role.

105) What is the cost of a dental education?

Without a doubt, dental school is very expensive. Although costs will vary, especially if you are at a state school vs. a private school, the best way to choose a school isn't based on cost of attendance. Although it will weigh heavily in your decision, it's important not to allow that to be the biggest decision. The overall average of a dental school education will range from $100,000 to almost over $300,000 depending on the school you choose to attend.

106) Will I receive ample patient contact if I am not in a city setting?

Ideally, a city setting will expose you to the most patients. However, since some schools are not in a city, they may have a shortage of patients. It is important to also see if you will be competing with post-doctorate students for patients. Although each school will give the chance to do the procedures, it is often difficult for schools in a rural setting to have additional patients for their dental students. The best way to find out about the clinical set up is to ask a current third or fourth-year student. Regardless, the majority of schools know how vital patient contact is for dental students and they make an effort to attract patients. Patients who need lots of dental work will flock to dental schools since the cost could be as low as a quarter of what they would pay a dentist in private practice. Many patients prefer the school setting, even though it may require additional time, since they know each student is being monitored by faculty members. For these individuals, there is a sense of trust when many people are diagnosing and are involved in the treatment.

107) How will the school of your choice assist a student having academic difficulty?

This is a tricky situation. Some schools will do everything to keep their students. Other schools will give you one chance and yet other schools will just dismiss students. The best thing to do is read the information packet you receive from the school. You should be able to find a section on academic policy. If you cannot find the schools' policy ask the dean. It is important to find out; some schools actually continue the weed-out process even once you are in dental school.

108) Will schools make accommodation for students with learning disabilities?

If you have a learning disability and it is documented, by law, you can request special consideration.

109) How are tests administered in dental schools?

Most of the schools have multiple choice tests. Some have written tests, and yet others will even have oral exams. It is also important to find out how the tests are administered. Does the school have a block exam policy? Do they give students time between exams? In addition, does the faculty keep the students in mind when preparing the exams? Every school has a different policy, so ask before you decide on the school! Some schools stagger their tests so you have time to study for each test; however it may be that you may have one test each week. Other schools may have a definite midterm and finals week where all your exams are given together. There are pros and cons to each. You just need to prepare and be organized throughout dental school.

110) Do people work while in dental school?

Dental school is a huge time commitment. However, if you are organized, there may be opportunity to work. Some dental schools offer research jobs, library jobs, and jobs on campus. This may provide some pocket change; however it is best to focus on school and graduating on time. If you have an opportunity to work with a dentist either on or off campus, that may be an excellent opportunity. But remember, your main priority is to succeed in dental school and learn as much as possible so you can be a competent dentist.

ஐ ൦ൠ

YOU GOT IN – NOW WHAT??

First and foremost, congratulations!!! It is time to celebrate and get excited about your future. You are one of the few people who got in to dental school this year. Here is a short checklist after you get that acceptance letter:

- ✓ Make sure to know when the deposit is due and mail it in as soon as possible. It is recommended to mail it in with signature verification.
- ✓ Start finding housing immediately. Do not wait for housing until the end, or you may be stuck with a bad deal or a bad location. Some schools will offer housing options but be your own advocate and research if this option is for you. It maybe well worth taking another trip down to the school and looking for more affordable and nicer housing.
- ✓ Visit the school once more, prior to matriculating. You can even bring your deposit with you. This is just to reassure yourself that you made the right decision.
- ✓ Start making connections with upper classmen. Get e-mails and phone numbers, and ask them any questions you may have. Ideally, talk to first-year students.
- ✓ Use social networking sites such as Facebook and Student Doctor Network® to get to know your classmates.
- ✓ Enjoy your summer prior to dental school. This is very important for those of you going straight to dental school from college. You need a break, and this maybe the longest break you get, other than retirement.
- ✓ Now is the time to learn basic dentistry. Go to the bookstore or borrow a textbook from a friend, and start getting familiar with the subjects such as Dental Anatomy.
- ✓ Familiarize yourself with the city you will be residing in.

- ✓ Move in at least two weeks before classes so you know your school and your colleagues.
- ✓ Most schools may introduce you with a 'big sib' or a upper classman who will guide you and may even give you their books notes. This maybe a gold mine worth of information. Always accept any help that is given from any upper classman. They may want to get rid of their notes or forget about their classes but for you this may make your life easier.
- ✓ If you do want to work during the summer before dental school work at a dental office. Try to absorb as much as possible about the new life you are going to embark on.
- ✓ As questions and keep an open mind.

This is a very exciting time! Follow the above tidbits and you will easily transition into dental school. Remember, your school and classmates are a family; you may have gotten through college independently, but that is a rare case in dental school. Dentistry is a profession that you need to rely on people and associate with people.

So, go give yourself a pat on the shoulder. You got in!

ಙ ಚ

DENTAL TERMINOLOGY

This part of the book is going to introduce you to basic dental terminology. Any profession has its own language, and the more comfortable you are with the terminology, the better you will be able to understand, communicate, and apply your knowledge. The terms here are going to help you during your interview and also during your first year of dental school. You may want to flip through the terms on the airplane or during a commercial break. It will help you get familiar with the dental lingo and may impress your interviewers and colleagues.

abscess: Any infections in the mouth, either in the soft tissue, bone, or tooth. An abscess can be seen radiographically or clinically.

alveolar bone: This is the bone that forms the "socket" that helps support the tooth into the jawbone. The bone surrounding the root of the tooth, anchoring it in place; loss of this bone is typically associated with severe periodontal (gum) disease.

amalgam: A common filling material used to repair cavities. The material, also known as "silver fillings," contains mercury in combination with silver, tin, copper, and sometimes zinc.

anaerobic bacteria: Bacteria that do not need oxygen to grow; they are generally associated with periodontal disease (gum disease).

analgesia: Something that causes pain relief.

anesthesia: A type of medication that results in partial or complete elimination of pain sensation; numbing a tooth is an example of local anesthesia; general anesthesia produces partial or complete unconsciousness for the patient.

antibiotic: A drug that inhibits or slows the growth of bacteria. Common antibiotics are penicillin, amoxicillin, and clindamycin.

antiseptic: An agent usually a chemical which can be applied to living tissues to kill bacteria. Listerine mouthwash is a common antiseptic.

apex: The tip of the root of a tooth. The nerve of the tooth exits from the apex and joins the main nerve of the region.

appliance: An appliance in dentistry could be a night guard, a retainer, or a denture. These usually are removable.

arch: There are two arches in the mouth. Maxillary arch is the top arch and the mandibular arch is the bottom arch.

baby bottle tooth decay (BBTD): Extreme and rampant decay commonly seen in infants and young children. Maxillary teeth are affected mainly due to continuous sweets given in a baby bottle. The sweet liquids cause the bacteria to continuously produce acid and slowly erode the teeth.

bicuspid a.k.a premolar: These are smaller than molars and have similar function of chewing and grinding. Most premolars have two cusps (bumps). Adults have eight premolars in their mouth or four in each arch, or two in each quadrant. Premolars are sometimes removed in order to make room to straighten teeth by orthodontics.

biopsy: Excision of suspicious tissue for pathological examination. Not all biopsies are excision of tissue. Some can be brushed (brush biopsy). Aspiration is also another method to send tissue to the lab for examination.

bite-wing: Another term for a single radiograph which shows in detail the *interproximal* areas (between teeth) and the supporting bone. Bite-wings do not show the root of the tooth.

bleaching: Chemical or laser treatment of natural teeth that uses peroxide to produce the whitening effect. Patients have many ways to whiten their teeth including strips, toothpaste, bleaching trays, and laser whitening.

bonding: The covering of a tooth surface with a tooth-colored composite to repair and/or change the color or shape of a tooth; for instance, due to stain or damage. Patients/dentists use bonding and composites interchangeably.

bone resorption: Decrease in the amount of bone supporting the roots of teeth; a common result of periodontal (gum) disease. Bone loss is started by poor hygiene, which leads to gingivitis (bleeding gums). If this is not reversed, then bone loss occurs due to the continued infection.

braces: Devices (bands, wires, ceramic appliances) put in place by orthodontists to gradually reposition teeth to a more favorable alignment. Now many cases can be completed with clear braces such as Invisalign®.

bridge: Stationary dental prosthesis (appliance) cemented/fixed to teeth adjacent to a space; replaces one or more missing teeth, cemented, or bonded to supporting teeth or implants adjacent to the space. A bridge is also called a fixed partial denture.

bruxism: Grinding or gnashing of the teeth, most commonly during sleep. Grinding teeth is a habit related to stress. It may be hereditary.

calcium: An element needed for the development of healthy teeth, bones, and nerves.

calculus: Hard, calcium-like deposits that form on teeth due to inadequate plaque control, often stained yellow or brown. Also known as "tartar."

canker sore: Sores or small shallow ulcers that appear in the mouth and often make eating and talking uncomfortable; they typically appear in people between the ages of 10 and 20 and last about a week in duration before disappearing. There are many theories about canker sores; most of them discuss stress, lowering of the immune system, and lack of iron or vitamins. Most people complain of cancer sores during high stress.

cap: Common term for a dental crown. Many patients will call a crown a "cap."

caries: Tooth decay or "cavities." When people say cavities they mean caries.

cementum: Hard tissue that covers the roots of teeth. The cementum joins the peridontial ligaments to the bone in the socket.

clasp: Device that holds a removable partial denture to stationary teeth. You may have seen metal hooks when people smile. Those are known as clasps on a partial denture. In other words clasps, clasp teeth. Clasps can be metal or acrylic (plastic).

cleaning: Removal of plaque and calculus (tarter) from teeth, generally above the gum line. In dentistry a cleaning is known as a prophylaxis or "prophy."

cleft lip: A physical split or separation of the two sides of the upper lip. This is due to the malformation of the lip/mouth during development.

cleft palate: A split or opening in the roof of the mouth. This is similar to a cleft lip, but the main malformation is inside the mouth on the palate.

composite resin filling: Tooth-colored restorative material composed of plastic with small glass or ceramic particles; usually "cured" or hardened with a curing light which sets the photosensitive materials in the composites. Composites are generally replacing unaesthetic metal fillings called amalgams.

conventional denture: A denture that is ready for placement in the mouth about two to three months after the teeth have been removed. Usually this is termed full denture and made for patients who are completely edentulous (having no teeth).

cosmetic (aesthetic) dentistry: A branch of the dental profession catering to improving the aesthetics of the smile.

crown: The portion of the tooth which is shown above the gum line (clinical crown) or a fabricated prosthesis which is cemented on a preparation. A common term for a crown is a "cap."

cuspids a.k.a canine: The third tooth from the center of the mouth, to the back of the mouth. Also known as canines, these are the fangs seen in animals at the front of the mouth, and are used to shear food. Note: a cuspid has one cusp, whereas a bicuspid has two cusps.

cusps: Pointed formations on teeth that help facilitate chewing.

cyst: An abnormal sac containing gas, fluid, or a semi-solid material.

D.D.S.: Doctor of Dental Surgery -- equivalent to D.M.D., Doctor of Dental Medicine. Many schools offer the D.D.S. degree upon graduation; however this is similar to the D.M.D. degree.

decay: Destruction of tooth structure caused by toxins, produced by bacteria. Decay is another synonym for cavities.

deciduous teeth: Commonly called "baby teeth" or primary teeth; the first set of (usually) 20 teeth.

demineralization: Loss of mineral from tooth enamel just below the surface in a carious lesion; usually appears as a white area on the tooth surface. Demineralization is the beginning of a cavity which sometimes can be reversed by applying fluoride or better oral hygiene.

dentin: Inner layer of tooth structure, immediately under the surface enamel. This is a yellow looking layer, softer than enamel.

denture: A removable replacement of artificial teeth for missing natural teeth and surrounding tissues. Complete dentures are for arches that are missing all of the teeth, partial dentures are for arches which have some natural teeth available and they are used for anchors of the dentures.

D.M.D.: Doctor of Medical Dentistry; equivalent to D.D.S., Doctor of Dental Surgery. Some schools give this degree which is the same as a D.D.S.

dry mouth: A condition in which the flow of saliva is reduced and there is not enough saliva to keep the mouth moist. There are many reasons for dry mouth. Most dry mouth is caused by medications and diseases such as Sjögren's syndrome. Excessive alcohol and tobacco can also cause dry mouth. The medical terminology for dry mouth is xerostomia.

dry socket: A painful occurrence after an extraction where there is a failure for a blood clot to form or has been dislodged. This is mainly caused by patient smoking or drinking alcohol after the procedure.

Patients are told to refrain from tobacco and alcohol for at least 72 hours after an extraction.

edentulous: When there are no teeth. This is an adjective describing the condition of the patient or certain areas of the mouth.

enamel: The hardest layer of the tooth which covers the entire clinical crown of a natural tooth. This is also the hardest tissue in the entire body.

endodontics: A specialty of dentistry which focuses on the dental pulp and root tissues. The term root canal or "endo" is used to describe a root canal therapy which is performed when the nerve of the tooth has been infected or compromised.

endodontist: A dental specialist that specializes on the dental pulp or the nerve of the tooth.

eruption: The entry of a tooth into the mouth.

extraction: Removal of a tooth.

filling: Replacing of lost tooth structure (mainly due to decay) with metal, porcelain, or resin materials.

fistula: A channel that leads an opening for pus to escape. Usually where an abscess occurs.

flossing: A thread-like material used to clean between the contact areas of teeth. Emphasis is placed on proper hygiene to prevent cavities between teeth.

fluoride: A mineral that helps strengthen teeth enamel. This is found in toothpaste, tap water, and can be applied by a dentist or hygienist to prevent decay.

fluorosis: Discoloration of enamel structure due to ingesting too much fluoride during tooth development. This is more of an esthetic issue. The teeth that have fluorosis are extremely resistant to tooth decay.

general dentist: The primary dental provider who encompasses all aspects of dental care. He or she can refer to a specialist for any case he or she thinks they cannot handle.

gingiva: Another term for gums.

gingivectomy: Surgical removal of gum tissue.

gingivitis: Inflamed and tender gum tissue that may bleed easily when touched or brushed. Gingivitis is caused by bad oral hygiene, stress, and hormonal changes. The most effective way to control it is proper oral hygiene. If not controlled over time, it can lead to periodontal disease which may cause loss of teeth.

gum recession: Loss of gum tissue on the roots due to abrasion, grinding, or crowding of teeth. These areas can be very sensitive to cold.

gutta percha: Rubbery material used in the filling of root canals.

halitosis: Bad breath.

handpiece: Another name for dental drill used to drill teeth. A high speed handpiece is used for fillings, crown preparations, etc. A slow speed can be used for endodontics, removing delicate areas of the tooth.

hard palate: Roof of the mouth.

hygienist: A licensed dental professional who works under the supervision of a dentist and mainly educates patients in proper oral hygiene and also does prophylaxis and scaling and root planning treatment.

hypersensitivity: When a tooth is sensitive abnormally to hot, cold, sweets, and acids.

immediate denture: A denture that is made in advance and placed at the same appointment when the teeth are removed. This denture needs more adjustments afterwards, but one benefit is that it gives the patient a new smile immediately.

impacted tooth: A tooth that has either not erupted due to its orientation in the bone, or has erupted partially. Impacted teeth can cause problems such as food impaction hence causing more decay, crowding, and pain. Most impacted teeth have to be removed surgically.

implant: A metal screw/rod that is placed into the jawbone, usually made up of biocompatible material such as titanium. After several months of healing, it fuses to the bone and then a crown is placed on the screw. Implants are great restorations for someone missing one or many teeth.

impression: A mold made of the mouth or specific area of the mouth.

incision and drainage: A surgical approach to alleviate swelling and drain the abscess of pus.

incisors: The four upper and lower front teeth. These teeth have no cusps, but incisal edges. As their name sounds, they are used for incising food.

inlay: A filling which usually is made out of ceramic. Instead of placing the filling the same day as a regular filling, an inlay maybe sent to a lab to be made. An inlay is between the cusps and usually is indicated when the size of the prep is too big for a conventional filling, but too small for a crown. An inlay involves less cutting of natural tooth structure than a crown.

malocclusion: mal- means bad. It is hence a bad bite or a bite that causes misalignment of the teeth or dental trauma.

mandible: The lower jaw.

maxilla: The upper jaw.

molars: Three back teeth in each dental quadrant used for grinding food. The wisdom teeth are called third molars. If you have all your wisdom teeth out, then you only have two molars per quadrant, or four per arch and eight in the total mouth.

mouth guard: A dental appliance which usually is fabricated with semi-soft plastic or resin. It sits on the teeth and prevents one from grinding or serves as protection from trauma (sports). Another name for a mouth guard is an occlusal guard.

muscle relaxant: A medication often prescribed to reduce stress, it is usually given to patients with jaw joint pain or to anxious patients.

nerve (root) canal: The dental pulp is the third tissue of a tooth after enamel and dentin. The pulp has nerves, lymphatics, and blood vessels. During a root canal, the nerve is removed and the space is sealed with gutta percha.

night guard: Similar to a mouth guard, this is also known as an occlusal guard. For patients who grind their teeth at night or during the day, this helps prevent damage to the remaining teeth.

nitrous oxide: A gas given to patients to reduce anxiety. This is also known as laughing gas.

NSAID: A non-steroidal anti-inflammatory drug, often used as a dental analgesic. This term may be used for ibuprofen. ASA may be used for aspirin.

occlusion: The relationship of the upper and lower teeth when the mouth is closed.

onlay: If the tooth needs a prosthesis bigger than a filling but smaller than a crown, then an onlay must be inserted. Similar to an inlay, the onlay is a big filling, but is fabricated by a dental lab and cemented into the preparation. They restore the tooth without compromising tooth much tooth structure. Onlays are sometimes called partial crowns. Onlays are bigger than inlays since a lot of the tooth structure is compromised and usually a cusp (or chewing surface) is lost due to fracture or decay.

oral cavity: Another name for the mouth. This includes the palate, teeth, gum, tongue, etc.

oral and maxillofacial radiologist: A specialty of dentistry where the main focus is to interpret and analyze radiographs of the oral maxillofacial region. The goal is to assess the complex tissue of the oral maxillofacial region for pathology and complicated diseases.

oral and maxillofacial surgery: Any surgery in the oral cavity which may include removing pathology, doing implants, or removing impacted teeth.

oral hygiene: Process of maintaining cleanliness of the teeth and related structures.

oral medicine: A specialty of dentistry where the goal is to manage medically complex patients.

oral pathologist: An oral health care provider who specializes in the study of oral pathology and disease of the oral cavity.

oral surgeon: A specialist in the dental profession who focuses in all types of surgery in the oral maxillofacial region.

orthodontics: A dental specialty where to goal is to correct malocclusion through the use of brackets and wires. The specialist who focuses only on correcting occlusion is called an orthodontist.

palate: Hard and soft tissue forming the roof of the mouth.

panoramic X-ray: A 2-Dimensional X-ray that shows the teeth and all the oral structures of the mouth including the jawbone, nerves, joints, sinuses, etc.

partial denture: A removable appliance that replaces some of the teeth.

pedodontics/pediatric dentistry: A dental specialty focusing on treatment of children, usually younger than 13.

periapical: Region at the end of the roots of teeth.

periapical X-rays: X-rays providing complete side views from the roots to the crowns of the teeth. Also known as a P.A.

periodontal ligament: Small fibers that connect the tooth to the jawbone. Also abbreviated PDL.

periodontist: The dental specialist who specializes in diagnosing, treating, and preventing diseases of the soft tissues of the mouth (the gums), as well as the supporting structures (bones) of the teeth.

periodontitis: An advanced stage of gum disease which usually starts with gingivitis and progresses to a point when the supporting structures that hold the teeth in place (gums, PDL, and bone) are destroyed.

permanent teeth: The teeth that replace the deciduous or primary teeth. Most adults have 32 teeth.

plaque: A whitish film that sticks on the teeth. If not brushed off, it gets harder and turns into calculus or tartar. Plaque is the main cause of gingivitis and decay.

pontic: The name of the tooth that is to be replaced on a bridge.

porcelain: A tooth-colored material that is heated in an oven and baked into a crown.

post: Usually a thick plastic or steel rod that is inserted into one of the canals that gives the remaining tooth strength to withstand chewing forces. A post is necessary if a tooth needs a crown but there is not enough tooth structure. Most teeth that need posts also have root canal therapy done.

pregnancy gingivitis: Tender and bleeding gums seen in patients who are pregnant. Main cause of gingivitis is plaque, but in pregnant women hormonal factors also cause gingivitis. Most pregnant women are told to brush and floss more frequently to prevent gingivitis and pregnancy tumors (inflamed tissue) due to food particles or plaque causing extreme growths.

primary teeth: The first set of 20 temporary teeth. Also called baby teeth, the primary dentition, or deciduous teeth.

prophylaxis: The cleaning of the teeth for the prevention of periodontal disease and tooth decay.

prosthetics: A fixed or removable appliance used to replace missing teeth (for example: bridges, partials, and dentures).

prosthodontist: A dental specialist who focuses on total mouth rehabilitation which may include crowns, dentures, and implants. A patient may be referred to a prosthodontist who may need to change their bite with prosthetics.

pulp: The third tissue in the tooth after enamel and dentin. The pulp has nerves, lymphatics, and blood.

radiographs: Another name for x-rays.

remineralization: Restoring enamel by ions which naturally occur in the saliva or topically by fluoride or calcium gels.

restorations: Any replacement for lost tooth structure such as fillings, inlays, onlays, crowns, bridges, implants, etc.

retainer: A removable appliance usually given after orthodontic therapy (braces) to keep the teeth from moving.

root: Part of the tooth which is submerged in the jawbone and keeps the tooth stable in the jaw.

root canal therapy: A procedure to save a tooth by removing the nerve. Usually a tooth has been infected or broken where the nerve or pulp has been compromised. If the nerve is not removed, intense pain is felt.

rubber dam: A latex barrier used to isolate the teeth and prevent contamination during a root canal or prevent any micro-instruments from being aspirated or swallowed by the patient.

saliva: A clear fluid produced by salivary glands which contains proteins, enzymes, and ions. Saliva is the main buffer in the mouth and helps re-mineralize the enamel on the teeth and also flush away plaque from the tooth surface.

salivary glands: Glands located in main areas of the mouth that produce saliva.

scaling and root planing: Also known as a deep cleaning. Unlike a normal prophylaxis, this cleaning requires the hygienist or dentist to remove plaque, tartar, and calculus from underneath the gums. Usually a patient is numb and scalers are used to scrape away the hard deposits from the root surfaces. Scaling is removing the buildup and planing is smoothing out the tooth surface.

sealants: A liquid resin that is applied in the grooves of the teeth to prevent cavities. It is ideal to place sealants as soon as molars/premolars erupt.

sedative: Any medication that is used to relax.

soft palate: The soft part of the palate that is located in the last third of the mouth.

space maintainer: A dental device hold the space of a tooth during a premature loss of a baby tooth.

supernumerary tooth: An extra tooth. Many people have more than 32 teeth. Any extra tooth is called a supernumerary tooth.

tartar: A common term for dental calculus. A very hard deposit which is very difficult to remove by brushing.

teething: Baby teeth pushing through gums. This is usually a period of discomfort for children.

temporomandibular joint (TMJ): The joints that hold the lower jaw (mandible). The joint not only rotates the jaw (open/closes) but also translates (comes out). Trauma or grinding, or not enough space for teeth may cause TMJ disorder which causes pain, popping, and clicking of the joint.

topical anesthetic: Ointment that produces mild anesthesia when applied to tissue surface. Orajel® in the stores is a topical anesthetic.

transplant: Placing a natural tooth in the empty socket of another tooth.

trauma: Any force which impacts the viability of a tooth or occlusion.

under bite: When the lower jaw comes out farther than the top jaw does.

veneer: Thin plates made of ceramic that are bonded to the front of the tooth for a more aesthetically-pleasing smile. Veneers are commonly used to close spaces, fix chipped teeth, and permanently whiten the smile.

wisdom teeth: The last teeth to erupt in the mouth, also called third molars. They usually erupt after age 18.

xerostomia: Another term for dry mouth which can be caused by auto-immune disease, prescription drugs, smoking, and/or drinking excessive alcohol.

ಏ ಙ

LIST OF DENTAL SCHOOLS IN THE UNITED STATES

Note: This list is current at the time of publication. It is highly recommended to contact the schools directly to get the proper contact information.

United States

Arizona School of Dentistry and Oral Health

Baylor College of Dentistry, A Member of The Texas A&M University System Health Science Center

Boston University, Goldman School of Dental Medicine

Case Western Reserve University School of Dentistry

Columbia University School of Dental and Oral Surgery

Harvard School of Dental Medicine

Howard University College of Dentistry

Loma Linda University School of Dentistry

Marquette University School of Dentistry

Medical College of Georgia School of Dentistry

Medical University of South Carolina College of Dental Medicine

New York University College of Dentistry

Nova Southeastern University College of Dental Medicine

Ohio State University College of Dentistry

Oregon Health & Science University School of Dentistry

Southern Illinois University School of Dental Medicine

State University of New York at Buffalo School of Dental Medicine

State University of New York at Stony Brook School of Dental Medicine

Temple University School of Dentistry

Tufts University School of Dental Medicine

University of Alabama at Birmingham School of Dentistry

University of California, Los Angeles School of Dentistry

University of California, San Francisco School of Dentistry

University of Colorado School of Dentistry

University of Connecticut School of Dental Medicine

University of Detroit Mercy School of Dentistry

University of Florida College of Dentistry

University of Illinois at Chicago College of Dentistry

University of Iowa College of Dentistry

University of Kentucky College of Dentistry

University of Louisville School of Dentistry

University of Maryland, Baltimore College of Dental Surgery

University of Medicine and Dentistry of New Jersey, New Jersey Dental School

University of Michigan School of Dentistry

University of Minnesota School of Dentistry

University of Mississippi School of Dentistry

University of Missouri-Kansas City School of Dentistry

University of Nebraska Medical Center, College of Dentistry

University of Nevada, Las Vegas School of Dental Medicine

University of North Carolina at Chapel Hill School of Dentistry

University of Oklahoma College of Dentistry

University of the Pacific School of Dentistry

University of Pennsylvania School of Dental Medicine

University of Pittsburgh School of Dental Medicine

University of Puerto Rico, School of Dentistry

University of Southern California School of Dentistry

University of Tennessee College of Dentistry

University of Texas Health Science Center at Houston Dental Branch

University of Texas Health Science Center at San Antonio Dental School

University of Washington School of Dentistry

Virginia Commonwealth University School of Dentistry

West Virginia University School of Dentistry

Canada

Dalhousie University Faculty of Dentistry

McGill University Faculty of Dentistry

University of Alberta Faculty of Dentistry

University of British Columbia Faculty of Dentistry

University Laval Faculty of Dentistry

University of Manitoba Faculty of Dentistry

University of Montreal Faculty of Dentistry

University of Saskatchewan College of Dentistry

University of Toronto Faculty of Dentistry

University of Western Ontario Faculty of Dentistry

ALABAMA

University of Alabama at Birmingham

Deadline Date: December 1
Telephone: (205) 934-3387
Fax: (205) 934-0209
E-mail: cindye@uab.edu
www.dental.uab.edu

Contact Person:

Cindy Edwards
Office of Admissions
University of Alabama at Birmingham
School of Dentistry
1530 3rd Avenue South, SDB 125
Birmingham, AL 35294-0007

Send materials only when the school or admissions officer contacts you.
- Application fee $50
- 2" x 2" photograph
- Supplemental application
- Transcripts

ARIZONA

Arizona School of Dentistry and Oral Health

Deadline Date: December 1
Telephone: (866) 626-2878 ext 2237
Fax: (660) 626-2969
E-mail: admissions@atsu.edu
www.atsu.edu

Contact Person:

> Donna Sparks
> Arizona School of Dentistry and Oral Health
> A.T. Still University
> 800 W Jefferson Street
> Kirksville, MO 63501

Send these materials to the dental school at the same time you send AADSAS materials:
- Official DAT scores

Send materials only when the school or admissions officer contacts you.
- Secondary application, due January 31
- Secondary application fee of $60

Midwestern University

> Deadline Date: January 1
> Telephone: (888) 247-9277
> Fax: (623) 572-3229
> E-mail: admissaz@midwestern.edu
> www.midwestern.edu/az-dental

Contact Person:

> James Walter
> Office of Admissions
> Midwestern University
> College of Dental Medicine
> 19555 N. 59th Avenue
> Glendale, AZ 85308

Send these materials to the dental school at the same time you send AADSAS materials:
- Official DAT scores from the ADA

- Send materials only when the school or admissions officer contacts you.
- Secondary application due March 6
- Secondary application fee $50

CALIFORNIA

Loma Linda University

Deadline Date: December 1
Telephone: (909) 558-4621 or (800) 422-4558
Fax: (909) 558-0195
E-mail: admissions_sd@llu.edu
www.dentistry.llu.edu

Contact Person:

Fred C. Kasrschke
Office of Admissions
Loma Linda University, Rm 5504
School of Dentistry
Loma Linda, CA 92350

Send materials only when the school or admissions officer contacts you.
- Supplemental application with fee
- Three letters of evaluation as specified in the supplementary application
- AADSAS official college/university transcript is fine until committee review; then official transcript needs to be sent.

University of California, Los Angeles

Deadline Date: January 1
Fax: (310) 825-9808
E-mail: dds_admissions@dentistry.ucla.edu
uclasod.dent.ucla.edu

Contact Person:

    Noemi Benitez
    University of California, Los Angeles
    School of Dentistry
    Office of Student Affairs & Outreach
    Room A0-111 CHS
    10833 LeConte Avenue
    Los Angeles, CA 90095-1762

Send these materials to the dental school at the same time you send AADSAS materials:
- Official DAT scores

Send materials only when the school or admissions officer contacts you.
- Application fee of $60
- Secondary application
- Official High School transcript (must be sent directly to the office, in addition to the copies submitted to AADSAS)
- Official undergraduate transcript(s) (must be sent directly to the office in addition to the copies submitted to AADSAS)

University of California, San Francisco

    Deadline Date: October 15
    Telephone: (415) 476-2737
    Fax: (415) 476-4226
    E-mail: admissions@dentistry.ucsf.edu
    dentistry.ucsf.edu

Contact Person:

    Office of Admissions
    University of California, San Francisco
    School of Dentistry
    513 Parnassus, Room S-619
    San Francisco, CA 94143-0430

Send materials only when the school or admissions officer contacts you:
- Application fee of $60 (U.S. citizens & permanent residents)
- Application fee of $80 (International students)
- UCSF supplemental application

University of Southern California

Deadline Date: February 1
Telephone: (213) 740-2841
Fax: (213) 740-8109
E-mail: uscsdadm@usc.edu
www.usc.edu/hsc/dental

Contact Person:

Sandra Bolivar
Office of Admissions and Student Affairs
University of Southern California
School of Dentistry
925 West 34th Street, Rm 201
Los Angeles, CA 90089-0641

Send these materials to the dental school at the same time you send AADSAS materials:
- Application fee of $85. Students requiring an I-20 for an F-1 student Visa must submit a $145 processing fee (send fee to: USC, School of Dentistry, File Number 12145-2, Los Angeles, CA 90074-2145)
- Official DAT scores

Send the following materials only when the school or admissions officer contacts you.
- 2" x 2" photograph

University of the Pacific Arthur A. Dugoni School of Dentistry

Deadline Date: December 1
Telephone: (415) 929-6491
Fax: (415) 749-3363
E-mail: SF_Admissions@pacific.edu
dental.pacific.edu

Contact Person:

Kathy Candito
Office of Student Services
University of the Pacific Arthur A. Dugoni
School of Dentistry
2155 Webster Street, Room 202
San Francisco, CA 94115

Send these materials to the dental school at the same time you send AADSAS materials:
- Application fee of $75
- Official DAT scores

Send these materials to the dental school only when an Admission Officer contacts you:
- Official transcripts

Western University of Health Sciences

Deadline Date: January 15
Telephone: (909) 469-5596
Fax: (909) 469-5570
E-mail: srowan@westernu.edu
www.westernu.edu

Contact Person:

Sean Rowan
Western University of Health Sciences
College of Dental Medicine

309 E Second Street
Pomona, CA 91766-1854

Send the following materials only when the school or admissions officer contacts you.
- Supplemental Application, which can be downloaded from website.
- Official DAT scores sent from the ADA

Send the following materials only when the school or admissions officer contacts you:
- Transcripts

COLORADO

University of Colorado

Deadline Date: January 1
Telephone: (303) 724-7120
Fax: (303) 724-7109
www.uchsc.edu/sod/

Contact Person:

Randy Kluender, DDS, MS
Admissions and Student Affairs
University of Colorado
School of Dental Medicine
13065 E. 17th Place
Mail Stop F833. PO Box 6508
Aurora, CO 80045

Send the following materials only when the school or admissions officer contacts you:
- Application fee of $50
- Verification of Colorado Residency Form
- Regent's questionnaire

CONNECTICUT

University of Connecticut

Deadline Date: January 15
Telephone: (860) 679-2175
Fax: (860) 679-1899
E-mail: robertson@nso2.uchc.edu
sdm.uchc.edu

Contact Person:

Dr. Edward Thibodeau
Office of Admissions, AGO30-MC3905
University of Connecticut
School of Dental Medicine
Farmington, CT 06030

Send these materials to the dental school at the same time you send AADSAS materials:
- Application fee of $75
- Official DAT scores

DISTRICT OF COLUMBIA

Howard University

Deadline Date: January 15
Telephone: (202) 806-0400
Fax: (202) 806-0354
www.howard.edu

Contact Person:

Dr. Cecile E. Skinner
Howard University
College of Dentistry
600 W Street, NW
Washington, DC 20059

Send the following materials only when the school or admissions officer contacts you.
- Application fee of $45
- Official college transcript(s)
- Official DAT scores
- Three letters of evaluation or a committee evaluation, if not previously submitted with AADSAS application

FLORIDA

Nova Southeastern University

Deadline Date: December 15
Telephone: (954)-262-1108 or (800) 356-0026 ext 1108
Fax: (954) 262-2282
E-mail: zarrett@nova.edu
www.nova.edu

Contact Person:

Su-Ann Zarrett
Nova Southeastern University
College of Dental Medicine
Enrollment Processing Services (EPS)
Attn: HPD/Dental Medicine
3301 College Avenue
PO Box 299000
Ft. Lauderdale, FL 33329-9905

Send these materials to the dental school at the same time you send AADSAS materials:
- Official DAT scores

Send these materials to the dental school only when an Admission Officer contacts you:
- Application fee of $50
- Supplemental application

University of Florida

Deadline Date: December 1
Telephone: (352) 273-5955
Fax: (352) 846-0311
E-mail: DMDadmissions@dental.ufl.edu
www.dental.ufl.edu

Contact Person:

Ms. Lauren Yuill
Office of Dental Admissions
University of Florida
College of Dentistry
PO Box 100445
Gainesville, FL 32610-0445

Send these materials to the dental school at the same time you send AADSAS materials:
- Official DAT Scores
- Send the following materials only when the school or admissions officer contacts you: Application fee of $30
- Supplemental formal Florida application

ILLINOIS

Southern Illinois University

Deadline Date: February 1
Telephone: (618) 474-7170
Fax: (618) 474-7249
E-mail: sdmapps@siue.edu
www.siue.edu/dentalmedicine

Contact Person:

Dr. Cornell Thomas

Office of Admissions and Records
Southern Illinois University
School of Dental Medicine
2800 College Avenue, Bldg 273
Room 2300
Alton, IL 62002-4798

Send these materials to the dental school at the same time you send AADSAS materials:
- Application fee of $20 (send check/money to Southern Illinois University (SIU/SDM) admissions with applicant's name)
- Official DAT scores
- Supplemental application
- Technical Standards Form from the website:
- www.siue.edu/dentalmedicine

University of Illinois at Chicago

Deadline Date: December 1
Telephone: (312) 996-1020
Fax: (312) 413-9050
E-mail: bespin1@uic.edu
dentistry.uic.edu

Contact Person:

Braulia Espinosa
University of Illinois at Chicago
College of Dentistry
Office of Student Admissions
801 S. Paulina M/C 621, Room 104
Chicago, IL 60612

Send these materials to the dental school at the same time you send AADSAS materials:
- Three letters of evaluation.

Send these materials to the dental school only when an Admission Officer contacts you:
- Application fee of $65 (do not submit your application fee until schools states they have received your AADSAS application.

INDIANA

Indiana University

Deadline Date: January 1
Telephone: (317) 274-5117
Fax: (317) 278-9066
Email: rkasberg@iupui.edu
www.iusd.iupui.edu

Contact Person:

Robert H. Kasberg Jr., Ph.D.
Office of Student Affairs
Indiana University
1121 W. Michigan Street, Room 130
Indianapolis, IN 46202-5186

Send these materials to the dental school only when an Admission Officer contacts you:
- Application fee of $50
- Application fee of $60 (International Students)

IOWA

University of Iowa

Deadline Date: November 1
Telephone: (319) 335-7157
Fax: (319) 335-7155
E-mail: elaine-brown@uiowa.edu
www.dentistry.uiowa.edu

Contact Person:

B. Elaine Brown
Student Affairs Office
University of Iowa
College of Dentistry
311 Dental Science Bldg North
Iowa City, IA 52242-1010

Send these materials to the dental school at the same time you send AADSAS materials:
- Official DAT scores from the ADA

Send these materials to the dental school only when an Admission Officer contacts you:
- Application fee of $60 (U.S. citizens and permanent residents)
- Application fee of $85 (International students)

KENTUCKY

University of Kentucky

Deadline Date: December 15
Telephone: (859) 323-6071
Fax: (859) 257-5550
E-mail: mlock2@email.uky.edu
www.mc.uky.edu/dentistry

Contact Person:

Melissa Lockard
Office of Admissions and Student Affairs
University of Kentucky
College of Dentistry
Chandler Medical Center
Room D-155
Lexington, KY 40536-0297

Send these materials to the dental school at the same time you send AADSAS materials:
- DAT scores

Send these materials to the dental school only when an Admission Officer contacts you:
- Application fee of $65

University of Louisville

Deadline Date: January 1
Telephone: (502) 852-5081
Fax: (502) 852-1210
E-mail: dmdadms@louisville.edu
www.louisville.edu/dental

Contact Person:

Robin Benningfield
Office of Admissions, Room 231
University of Louisville
School of Dentistry
501 S. Preston Street
Louisville, KY 40292-0001

Send these materials to the dental school at the same time you send AADSAS materials:
- Official DAT scores
- Send letters of recommendation directly to AADSAS including: Three letters of evaluation (two basic science professors and one personal reference). A committee letter is accepted as well.

Send these materials to the dental school only when an Admission Officer contacts you: Application fee of $50

MARYLAND

University of Maryland

Deadline Date: January 1
Telephone: (410) 706-7472
Fax: (410) 706-0945
E-mail: ddsadmissions@dental.umaryland.edu
www.dental.umaryland.edu

Contact Person:

Office of Admissions
University of Maryland
Baltimore College of Dental Surgery
6th Floor South – Room 6410
650 West Baltimore Street
Baltimore, MD 21201

Send these materials to the dental school at the same time you send AADSAS materials:
- Application fee of $75
- Official DAT scores

Send these materials to the dental school only when an Admission Officer contacts you:
- Supplemental application
- Recommendations letters from committee or from two-science faculty

MASSACHUSETTS

Boston University Goldman School of Dental Medicine

Deadline Date: February 1
Telephone: (617) 638-4787
Fax: (617) 638-4798
E-mail: sdmadmis@bu.edu

dentalschool.bu.edu

Contact Person:

Boston University Goldman School of Dental Medicine
Office of Admissions & Student Affairs
100 E. Newton Street, G305
Boston, MA 02118

Send these materials to the dental school at the same time you send AADSAS materials:
- Official DAT Scores sent by the ADA
- Official Canadian Dental Association scores sent by the CDA

Send these materials to the dental school only when an Admission Officer contacts you:
- Application fee of $65 (U.S. Citizens and Permanent Residence)
- Application fee of $95 (International applicants)

Harvard School of Dental Medicine

Deadline Date: December 15
Telephone: (617) 432-1443
Fax: (617) 432-3881
Email: hsdm_admissions@hsdm.harvard.edu
www.hsdm.harvard.edu/asp-html/

Contact Person:

Anne L. Berg
Office of Dental Education
Harvard School of Dental Medicine
188 Longwood Avenue
Boston, MA 02115

Send these materials to the dental school at the same time you send AADSAS materials:
- Application fee of $75
- Official DAT scores

Send these materials to the dental school only when an Admission Officer contacts you:
- 2" x 2" photograph (if invited for interview)
- High school transcript (if invited for interview)

Tufts University

Deadline Date: February 1
Telephone: (617) 636-6639
Fax: (617) 636-0309
E-mail: denadmissions@tufts.edu
www.dental.tufts.edu

Contact Person:

Melissa L. Bradbury
Office of Admissions
Tufts University
School of Dental Medicine
One Kneeland Street, 7th floor
Boston, MA 02111

Send these materials to the dental school at the same time you send AADSAS materials:
- Official DAT scores

Send these materials to the dental school only when an Admission Officer contacts you: Application fee of $60

MICHIGAN

University of Michigan

Deadline Date: December 1
Telephone: (734) 763-3316
E-mail: ddsadmissions@umich.edu
www.dent.umich.edu

Contact Person:

Dr. Marilyn W. Woolfolk
Patricia A. Katcher
Predoctoral Admissions
The University of Michigan
School of Dentistry - G226
1011 N. University Avenue
Ann Arbor, MI 48109-1078

Send these materials to the dental school at the same time you send AADSAS materials:
- Application fee of $50
- Official DAT scores
- 2" x 2" photograph (optional)

University of Detroit Mercy

Deadline Date: February 1
Telephone: (313) 494-6611 or (313) 494-6650
Fax: (313) 494-6659
E-mail: dental@udmercy.edu
www.dental.udmercy.edu

Contact Person:

Karin A. LaRose-Neil (MB 38)
University of Detroit Mercy
School of Dentistry
Office of Admissions, MB 38

2700 Martin Luther King Jr. Boulevard
Detroit, MI 48208-2576

Send these materials to the dental school at the same time you send AADSAS materials:
- Application fee of $75
- 2" x 2" signed photograph
- Official DAT score
- Official transcripts from all colleges/universities attended

Canadian Applicants
- High school transcripts

International Applicants
- Course-By-Course Evaluation Report prepared by the Education Credential Evaluators, Inc.
- Official TOEFL IBT results (100 total/25 each section)
- Official U.S. college/university transcript for one year of academic study (32 semester hours)

MINNESOTA

University of Minnesota

Deadline Date: December 1
Telephone: (612) 625-7477
Fax: (612) 624-0882
E-mail: ddsapply@umn.edu
www.dentistry.umn.edu

Contact Person:

Office of Admissions and Diversity
University of Minnesota
School of Dentistry
15-163 Malcolm Moos Hlth Sci. Twr
515 Delaware Street, SE
Minneapolis, MN 55455-0329

Send these materials to the dental school at the same time you send AADSAS materials:
- Application fee of $75
- Two letters of evaluation from science faculty and one from an employer
- UM School of Dentistry supplemental application
- Official DAT scores
- Official TOEFL scores for all non-native English speakers
- 2" x 2" photograph required

MISSOURI

University of Missouri - Kansas City

Deadline Date: October 1
Telephone: (816) 235-2080
Fax: (816) 235-2157
E-mail: dds@umkc.edu
dentistry.umkc.edu

Contact Person:

Richie Bigham
Office of Student Programs
University of Missouri-Kansas City
School of Dentistry
650 East 25th Street, Room 420
Kansas City, MO 64108-2784

Send these materials to the dental school at the same time you send AADSAS materials:
- Application fee $45
- Official DAT scores
- The UMKC School of Dentistry Application Survey
- 2" x 2" photograph

NEBRASKA

Creighton University

Deadline Date: February 1
Telephone: (800) 544-5072 or (402) 280-2695
Fax: (402) 280-5094
E-mail: denschadm@creighton.edu
cudental.creighton.edu

Contact Person:

Creighton University
School of Dentistry
Admissions Office
2500 California Plaza
Omaha, NE 68178

Send these materials to the dental school at the same time you send AADSAS materials:
- Application fee of $45
- Supplemental Application
- Official DAT scores
- Photograph

University of Nebraska

Deadline Date: February 1
Telephone: (402) 472-1363 or (800) 332-0265
Fax: (402) 472-5290
E-mail: gmcanfie@unmc.edu
www.unmc.edu/dentistry

Contact Person:

Glenda Canfield
Office of Admissions
University of Nebraska Medical Center
College of Dentistry

40th and Holdrege Street
Lincoln, NE 68583-0740

Send these materials to the dental school at the same time you send AADSAS materials:
- Application fee of $50
- Small photograph
- Official DAT scores

NEVADA

University of Nevada, Las Vegas

Deadline Date: January 1
Telephone: (702) 774-2520
Fax: (702) 774-2521
E-mail: UNLVDentSch@unlv.edu
dentalschool.unlv.edu

Contact Person:

Dr. Christine C. Ancajas
University of Nevada, Las Vegas
School of Dental Medicine
1001 Shadow Lane
MS 7411
Las Vegas, NV 89106-4124

Send these materials to the dental school at the same time you send AADSAS materials:
- Application fee of $50 (payable to Board of Regents - cashier's check or money order)
- Official DAT scores
- Supplemental application (may be downloaded from website)
- 2" x 2" color photograph

NEW JERSEY

University of Medicine and Dentistry of New Jersey

Deadline Date: December 1
Telephone: (973) 972-5362
Fax: (973) 972-0309
E-mail: armandsa@umdnj.edu
dentalschool.umdnj.edu

Contact Person:

Jeffrey Linfante, DMD
Sandie Armand
Office of Admissions and Student Recruitment
University of Medicine and Dentistry of New Jersey
Room B830
110 Bergen Street
Newark, NJ 07101-1709

Send these materials to the dental school at the same time you send AADSAS materials:
- Application fee of $75

NEW YORK

Columbia University College of Dental Medicine

Deadline Date: January 16
Telephone: (212) 305-3478
Fax: (212) 305-1034
E-mail: jmm10@columbia.edu
dental.columbia.edu

Contact Person:

Joseph McManus, DMD
Office of Admissions and Student Affairs
Columbia University College of Dental Medicine

630 West 168th Street
New York, NY 10032

Send these materials to the dental school at the same time you send AADSAS materials:
- Application fee of $75
- Official DAT scores

New York University

Deadline Date: February 1
Telephone: (212) 998-9818
Fax: (212) 995-4240
E-mail: dental.admissions@nyu.edu
www.nyu.edu/dental

Contact Person:

Eugenia E. Mejia, Ph.D
Office of Student Affairs and Admissions
New York University
345 East 24th Street, Rm 10 W
New York, NY 10010-9818

Send these materials to the dental school at the same time you send AADSAS materials:
- Application processing fee of $75
- Official DAT scores

Send these materials to the dental school only when an Admission Officer contacts you:
- 2" x 2" color photograph
- Supplemental application

University at Buffalo

Deadline Date: December 1
Telephone: (716) 829-2839

Fax: (716) 833-3517
E-mail: ub-sdm-admissions@buffalo.edu
www.sdm.buffalo.edu

Contact Person:

Dr. Robert B. Joynt
Academic and Student Affairs
University at Buffalo
School of Dental Medicine
315 Squire Hall
Buffalo, NY 14214

Send these materials to the dental school at the same time you send AADSAS materials:
- Application fee of $50
- Official DAT scores

Stony Brook University

Deadline Date: January 15
Telephone: (631) 632-3745
Fax: (631) 632-7130
E-mail: patricia.berry@stonybrook.edu
www.hsc.stonybrook.edu/dental

Contact Person:

Dr. Debra Cinotti
Office of Admissions and Student Affairs
Stony Brook University
School of Dental Medicine
Rockland Hall, Rm 115
Stony Brook, NY 11794-8709

Send these materials to the dental school at the same time you send AADSAS materials:
- Application fee of $75
- Official college transcript

NORTH CAROLINA

University of North Carolina at Chapel Hill

Deadline Date: November 1
Telephone: (919) 966-4565
Fax: (919) 966-5796
E-mail: ad_guckes@dentistry.unc.edu
www.dent.unc.edu

Contact Person:

Dr. Albert Guckes
Office of Academic Affairs
University of North Carolina at Chapel Hill
School of Dentistry
1050 Old Dental Bldg, CB #7450
Chapel Hill, NC 27599-7450

Send these materials to the dental school at the same time you send AADSAS materials:
- Supplemental application
- https://www.dent.unc.edu/secure/academic/programs/dds/apps/
- Supplemental Processing fee of $78

OHIO

Case School of Dental Medicine

Deadline Date: January 1
Telephone: (216) 368-2460
Fax: (216) 368-3204
E-mail: dentadmit@po.cwru.edu
dental.case.edu/

Contact Person:

David A. Dalsky

Office of Admissions
Case School of Dental Medicine
School of Dental Medicine
10900 Euclid Avenue
Cleveland, OH 44106-4905

Send these materials to the dental school at the same time you send AADSAS materials:
- Application fee of $45
- Official DAT scores

The Ohio State University

Deadline Date: September 15
Telephone: (614) 292-3361
Fax: (614) 292-0813
E-mail: dentadmit@osu.edu
www.dent.osu.edu/admissions/

Contact Person:

Recruitment and Admissions
The Ohio State University
College of Dentistry - #195
305 West 12th Avenue
Rm 0114 Postle Hall
Columbus, OH 43218-2357

Send these materials to the dental school at the same time you send AADSAS materials:
- Application fee of $60 (U.S. Permanent Residents)
- Application fee of $70 (International students)
- Supplemental application
- DAT scores
- Observation of Offices Report & Community Service Report (both reports are located at www.dent.ohio-state.edu/admissions

OKLAHOMA

University of Oklahoma

Deadline Date: September 1
Telephone: (405) 271-3530
Fax: (405) 271-3423
E-mail: dentistry-admissions@ouhsc.edu
dentistry.ouhsc.edu

Contact Person:

Sally Davenport
Office of Student Affairs
University of Oklahoma
College of Dentistry
1201 N. Stonewall Avenue, Room 512
Oklahoma City, OK 73117-1214

Send these materials to the dental school at the same time you send AADSAS materials:
- Application supplemental and fee of $65
- Official DAT scores
- Recommendation from a dentist

OREGON

Oregon Health and Science University

Deadline Date: November 1
Telephone: (503) 494-5274
Fax: (503) 494-6244
E-mail: sodadmit@ohsu.edu
www.ohsu.edu/sod

Contact Person:

Mark D. Mitchell
Office of Admissions and Student Affairs

Oregon Health and Science University
School of Dentistry
611 SW Campus Drive, Rm 214
Portland, OR 97239-3097

Send these materials to the dental school at the same time you send AADSAS materials:
- Application fee of $75
- Official DAT scores

PENNSYLVANIA

The Maurice H. Kornberg School of Dentistry, Temple University

Deadline Date: February 1
Telephone: (215) 707-7663 or (800) 441-4363
E-mail: jeremy.hull@temple.edu
www.temple.edu/dentistry

Contact Person:

Office of Admissions and Student Affairs
The Maurice H. Kornberg School of Dentistry
Temple University
3223 North Broad Street
Philadelphia, PA 19140

Send these materials to the dental school only when an Admission Officer contacts you:
- Application fee of $30

University of Pennsylvania

Deadline Date: January 1
Telephone: (215) 898-8943
Fax: (215) 898-5243
E-mail: dental-admissions@pobox.upenn.edu

www.dental.upenn.edu

Contact Person:

Corky Cacas
Office of Admissions
Robert Schattner Center
University of Pennsylvania
School of Dental Medicine
240 South 40th Street
Philadelphia, PA 19104-6030

Send these materials to the dental school at the same time you send AADSAS materials:
- Application fee of $50
- Supplemental application
- Official DAT Scores

University of Pittsburgh

Deadline Date: December 1
Telephone: (412) 648-8437
Fax: (412) 648-9571
E-mail: mangold@pitt.edu
www.dental.pitt.edu

Contact Person:

Dr. Kenneth Etzel
University of Pittsburgh
School of Dental Medicine
Recruitment/Financial Office
3501 Terrace Street, Rm 2114
Pittsburgh, PA 15261-1945

Send these materials to the dental school at the same time you send AADSAS materials:
- Processing fee of $35

- Processing fee of $50 (International students)
- 2" x 2" recent photograph
- Official DAT scores
- Letters of evaluation if not sent to AADSAS

PUERTO RICO

University of Puerto Rico

Deadline Date: December 1
Telephone: (787) 758-2525 ext 5228 and 5212
Fax: (787) 282-7117
E-mail: cmenendez@rcm.upr.edu or rvelez@rcm.upr.edu
www.upr.clu.edu

Contact Person:

Carmen Menendez
Office of Admissions
University of Puerto Rico
School of Dentistry
Medical Sciences Campus
PO Box 365067, Room 201
San Juan, PR 00936-5067

Send these materials to the dental school at the same time you send AADSAS materials:
- Application fee of $15
- Official college transcript for all colleges attended
- 2" x 2" photograph
- Official DAT scores
- Two letters of evaluation

SOUTH CAROLINA

Medical University of South Carolina

Deadline Date: December 1
Telephone: (843) 792-4892
Fax: (843) 792-6615
E-mail: linerw@musc.edu
www.musc.edu/em

Contact Person:

Bill Liner
Medical University of South Carolina
College of Dental Medicine
Office of Enrollment Management
41 Bee Street
PO Box 250203
Charleston, SC 29425-2970

Send these materials to the dental school at the same time you send AADSAS materials:
- Application fee of $75 (submit online with supplemental application, available July 1)
- Supplemental application
- Official college transcript for all colleges attended
- Official DAT scores from the ADA
- Confidential committee evaluation

TENNESSEE

Meharry Medical College

Deadline Date: January 15
Telephone: (615) 327-6223
E-mail: admissions@mmc.edu
www.mmc.edu

Contact Office:

> Allen D. Mosley
> Meharry Medical College
> School of Dentistry
> Office of Admissions and Records
> 1005 Dr. D.B. Todd Jr. Blvd
> Nashville, TN 37208

Send these materials to the dental school At the Same Time you send AADSAS materials:
- Supplemental application
- Official DAT scores
- 2 x 2 inch photograph with your name and AADSAS ID # on the back

TEXAS

Baylor College of Dentistry

> Deadline Date: October 1
> Telephone: (214) 828-8231
> Fax: (214) 874-4521
> E-mail: admissions-bcd@bcd.tamhsc.edu
> www.bcd.tamhsc.edu

Contact Person:

> Office of Recruitment and Admissions
> Baylor College of Dentistry
> Texas A&M Health Science Center
> 3302 Gaston Avenue
> Dallas, TX 75246

Send these materials to the dental school at the same time you send AADSAS materials:
- Application fee $35
- DAT scores

- Non-Texas residents must submit a BCD paper application (available on www.bcd.tamhsc.edu)

Note: If you are a Texas resident and are applying to Texas dental schools, you MUST apply through the Texas Medical and Dental Application Service (TMDSAS).

University of Texas Health Science Center at Houston

Deadline Date: October 1
Telephone: (713) 500-4151
Fax: (713) 500-4425
E-mail: celeste.i.rivera@uth.tmc.edu or utdds@uth.tmc.edu
www.uth.tmc.edu

Contact Person:

Celeste I. Rivera
Office of Student and Alumni Affairs
University of Texas Health Science Center at Houston
Dental Branch
6516 M.D. Anderson Blvd, Suite 155
Houston, TX 77030

Send these materials to the dental school at the same time you send AADSAS materials:
- Health Professions Committee Evaluation
- Photograph

Send these materials to the dental school only when an Admission Officer contacts you:
- Transcripts
- DAT scores
- Photograph

University of Texas Health Science Center at San Antonio

Deadline Date: October 1
Telephone: (210) 567-2674

Fax: (210) 567-2645
E-mail: dsprospect@uthscsa.edu
www.uthscsa.edu

Contact Person:

Sofia C. Montes
University of Texas Health Science Center at San Antonio
Dental School
7703 Floyd Curl Drive, MSC 7702
San Antonio, TX 78229-3900

Send these materials to the dental school only when an Admission Officer contacts you:
- Supplemental Application

Note: Texas residents applying to the Texas dental schools MUST apply through the Texas Medical and Dental Schools Application Service (TMDSAS). Non-Texas residents applying through AADSAS should NOT submit a second application through TMDSAS.

VIRGINIA

Virginia Commonwealth University

Deadline Date: November 1
Telephone: (804) 828-9196
Fax: (804) 828-5288
E-mail: mhealy@vcu.edu
www.dentistry.vcu.edu

Contact Person:

Dr. Michael Healy
Virginia Commonwealth University
School of Dentistry
PO Box 980566
Richmond, VA 23298-0566

Send these materials to the dental school at the same time you send AADSAS materials:
- Application fee of $70
- Official DAT scores
- 2" x 2" passport photograph

Send these materials to the dental school only when an Admission Officer contacts you: VCU Supplemental application form (only candidates selected for interview)

WASHINGTON

University of Washington

Deadline Date: November 1
Telephone: (206) 543-5840
Fax: (206) 616-2612
E-mail: askuwsod@u.washington.edu
www.dental.washington.edu

Contact Person:

Kathleen Craig
Office of Student Services
Admissions & Outreach
University of Washington
School of Dentistry
Rm HSB D323
Box 356365
Seattle, WA 98195-6365

Send these materials to the dental school only when an Admission Officer contacts you:
- Application fee of $35
- Transcripts
- Supplemental application
- Letters of evaluation

WEST VIRGINIA

West Virginia University

Deadline Date: November 1
Telephone: (304) 293-3522
Fax: (304) 293-8561
E-mail: susie.brown@mail.wvu.edu
www.hsc.wvu.edu/sod/index.html

Contact Person:

Susan Brown
Office of Dental Admissions and Records
West Virginia University
School of Dentistry
Robert C. Byrd Health Science Center
1170 Health Science N
PO Box 9815
Morgantown, WV 26506-9815

Send these materials to the dental school at the same time you send AADSAS materials:
- Official DAT scores

Send these materials to the dental school only when an Admission Officer contacts you:
- Application fee of $50

WISCONSIN

Marquette University

Deadline Date: February 1
Telephone: (800) 445-5385
Fax: (414) 288-6505
E-mail: brian.trecek@marquette.edu
www.marquette.edu/dentistry

Contact Person:

Brian Trecek
Marquette University
School of Dentistry
PO Box 1881
Milwaukee, WI 53201-1881

Send these materials to the dental school at the same time you send AADSAS materials:
- Application fee of $45
- Official DAT scores

ಐ ೧ಽ

FINANCING YOUR DENTAL EDUCATION

It is no doubt that dental school is rigorous, but it's also expensive. Every year, dental school tuition is going up faster than inflation. The demand for dentists is growing due to the exponential increase in population and the increasing amount of current dentists retiring. Every year about 6,000 dentists are retiring, and only a little over 4,000 are entering into the job market.

Regardless of how promising this sounds, your investment in dentistry will be one of the most expensive investments of time and money you will make in your life. In this chapter, our goal is going to be to go over some basics so you can go to dental school and accrue the least amount of debt possible.

First and foremost, make sure you try to pay off all of your consumer debt prior to entering dental school. That means your credit cards, your car, or other loans you've made with family members or friends. Avoid getting tangled in more debt outside of tuition and living expenses. Loan companies may entice you to borrow more than needed, but keep it at the minimum. Most schools will give you a detailed expense list as well as the average expenses for living. Usually these figures are more than enough, or even sometimes exaggerated to make sure students know what to pay. The figure that is not exaggerated is the cost of tuition. The school will have a set tuition and it will tell you exactly it wants out of you. Your living budget is up to you.

First, you want to know how much debt you have before going to dental school. If you have undergraduate debt, you can figure out your debt by going to the National Loan Data System (NSLDS) at www.nslds.ed.gov. Next you want to maintain exceptional credit before dental school and during dental school. Things will just get harder with bad credit. So pay your bills on time, keep a watch on expenditures, and do not sign up for things that will cause you to default on payment like magazines, Internet, or music clubs. Check your credit and know your FICO® score. The FICO® score can be obtained by going to www.myfico.com

Once you choose a dental school, talk to your financial advisor. Usually, every dental school has one and they are available to discuss the tuition and other expenses. Once you establish where you are going to live, you can develop an ideal shell of expenses. Any unnecessary expense needs to be thrown out. Defer your student loans that you have previously by contacting your school or loan processor. Remember, financial aid is not a scholarship and needs to be paid back. Also, financial aid will only pay a student what the school has determined to be basic costs such as tuition, books, living expenses, and food.

In the next section, we'll discuss the two major costs associated with dental school: direct costs and indirect costs.

Direct costs consist of your education, which include tuition and books. Indirect costs are costs that are not part of your education, but needed nonetheless because sleeping in the library is not going to be an option. Indirect costs are room and board, transportation (recommended not to have a car), travel, and food.

The school will provide all accepted candidates with a Cost of Attendance sheet. This is just a summary of what the school expects the student to deal with each year. Remember, this is just an estimate. Tuition, fees, and books remain consistent on the Cost of Attendance sheet, but the indirect costs may vary. Your goal should be to be lower than what the Cost of Attendance sheets states. For example, if the school has placed $12,000 per year for rent, it usually means your rent should be less than $1,000 a month. Most schools will only use the months you are actively participating in studying. So, for the first year if you are only in school for nine months then they will calculate that for nine months. If rent is estimated at $12,000, then that means it is for nine months, which is estimating $1,333 a month. However, usually leases are for one year. So if you get a loan for $12,000 and your lease is $1,333 a month you will actually need $15,996 for your room. If you know that your loan is based on the Cost of Attendance sheet, then be aware it is based on the months you are *actively* engaging in school. There are ways to increase your loan but they are cumbersome and most likely you will either need to borrow money from family members or take on private loans which usually have very astronomical interest rates.

Also, understand some state schools that get funding from the state will have big differences in tuition costs for in-state residents versus those who come from out of state. Some schools have provisions for out of state applicants to become in-state residents after one year, usually if they purchase a home in the state.

Funding your dental endeavors:

There are not many students who can afford to pay tuition out right. If you are, then you are very lucky. For the rest of us, there are many options available to help fund our education.

Let's talk about loans for dental students:

Stafford Loans: Direct/FFELP: These are the main loans most dental students use for dental education and possibly their undergraduate education. These are government loans. Parts of the loans are subsidized and the other part is unsubsidized. Subsidized loans mean that the interest is not accruing during your education. However, unsubsidized loans do accrue interest while you are studying.

For dental students, Health Professions Student Loans (HPSL) are made available. These loans are given based on financial need. You need not apply for them; instead, each school will review the FAFSA information and assess if you are eligible for the HPSL loan. The interest rate is 5% and there is a 12-month grace period after stopping your education. The criterion for this is that you need to be a citizen of the U.S. or a permanent resident. These loans are low interest loans.

Perkins Loans: This is a federal loan based on "exceptional" financial need. There is no need to apply, but instead the school will use your financial information to determine eligibility. Then, the government will either give you the loan directly to you or apply it to your schools charges. These are subsidized loans with a grace period and minimum interest rate.

Military Scholarships: Each branch of the military actively looks for dentists to join. They offer full scholarships with a stipend for living expenses for each year you receive their assistance. You will repay the military by serving in the armed forces for each year of assistance you received. There is a great benefit to this, since you can graduate without any debt. All tuition expenses and books are paid for.

National Health Service Corps (NHSC): Similar to the armed forces, the NHSC gives two or four-year scholarships with an agreement that you will serve in an underserved area in the United States. These scholarships are given by the U.S. Department of Health and Human Services.

Private Loans: These loans are the last resort and may cost you much more since their interest rates are much higher. Any bank or loan company, such as Sallie Mae or CitiBank provide these loans.

If you do need to get loans, the first thing you will need to do is fill out a FAFSA form which is available on www.fafsa.ed.gov. Each school usually requires candidates to fill this out for their assessment. Just because you are given a loan does not mean you have to accept all of it. If you know your need for living will only be $8,000 and you were given $12,000, then you can decline the loan and request only $8,000. Also understand that there are grace periods, but it is very important to pay off your loans on time. If you can, it is better to pay off more in the beginning, since majority of the loan is interest.

During your dental school years, you may be given the option to consolidate your loans. Consolidating allows you to merge your federal loans and may offer lower interest rates, one lender (and one bill), and could possibly reduce your monthly payments. You can learn more about loan consolidation by visiting www.loanconsolidation.ed.gov.

Here are some ways to help you save money during your education:

- ✓ Learn how to cook and eat at home.
- ✓ Take a lunch with you to school so you do not overspend.
- ✓ Before going out, research the venue and make a budget so you do not overspend.
- ✓ Buy used books or even better, borrow books.
- ✓ Buy a solid computer with insurance so you can have it for the entire four years.
- ✓ Participate in cheap entertainment on the school's campus or go see a movie (make sure to use your student id for an added discount)
- ✓ Join student club memberships, such as studentuniverse.com which give cheap deals to students.
- ✓ Clip coupons and buy things on sale.
- ✓ Make a shopping list and stick to it.

ಙ ಛ

Here is a worksheet for you to use as you research schools and figure out which school will be the best financial option for you.

School Name: _____

Tuition _____

School Fees _____

Books _____

Computer _____

Health Insurance _____

Rent (monthly payment for housing) _____

Food (calculate weekly average x4 x12) _____

Internet (calculate x 12) _____

Cable (calculate x 12) _____

Entertainment _____

Transportation _____

Grooming / Uniform _____

TOTAL: _____

School Name: _____

Tuition _____

School Fees _____

Books _____

Computer _____

Health Insurance _____

Rent (monthly payment for housing) _____

Food (calculate weekly average x4 x12) _____

Internet (calculate x 12) _____

Cable (calculate x 12) _____

Entertainment _____

Transportation _____

Grooming / Uniform _____

TOTAL: _____

School Name: _____

Tuition _____

School Fees _____

Books _____

Computer _____

Health Insurance _____

Rent (monthly payment for housing) _____

Food (calculate weekly average x4 x12) _____

Internet (calculate x 12) _____

Cable (calculate x 12) _____

Entertainment _____

Transportation _____

Grooming / Uniform _____

TOTAL: _____

School Name: _____

Tuition _____

School Fees _____

Books _____

Computer _____

Health Insurance _____

Rent (monthly payment for housing) _____

Food (calculate weekly average x4 x12) _____

Internet (calculate x 12) _____

Cable (calculate x 12) _____

Entertainment _____

Transportation _____

Grooming / Uniform _____

TOTAL: _____

FOR INTERNATIONAL DENTAL CANDIDATES

If you are a foreign-trained dentist, you most likely will have to continue some studies in the U.S. Foreign-trained dentists will have to go back to dental school for their clinical years -- there are only certain schools that have Advanced Standing Programs. With huge shortages of dentists, some states are allowing foreign-trained dentists to practice after they pass the boards and have done at least one year of General Practice Residency (GPR). However, it is up to the candidate to research which states are allowing this option. Each year, new rules and regulations develop and it is necessary to investigate by directly communicating with the dental board of each state.

Here are the minimum requirements for most U.S. Advanced Standing Schools:

- ✓ Have a dental degree from a foreign dental school
- ✓ Have your GPA converted/translated into English
- ✓ Pass English proficiency exams (TOEFL)
- ✓ Pass National Board Dental Examination Part I (NBDE I)

৪০ ৫৪

DENTAL SCHOOLS WITH ADVANCED STANDING PROGRAMS

Here is a list of dental schools with Advanced Standing Programs. Please contact the schools independently since these programs are very competitive and many schools change their requirements each year.

California

Loma Linda University School of Dentistry
Dental School
Loma Linda, CA 92350
Phone: (909) 558-4222
www.llu.edu/llu/dentistry

University of California at Los Angeles School of Dentistry
Center for Health Science
Rm 53-038
Los Angeles, CA 90095
Phone: (310) 206-6063
www.dent.ucla.edu

University of Southern California School of Dentistry
925 W. 34th Street
Los Angeles, CA 90089
Phone: (213) 740-2851
www.usc.edu/hsc/dental

University of California at San Francisco School of Dentistry
513 Parnassus Ave, S-630
San Francisco, CA 94143
Phone: (415) 476-1323
www.ucsf.edu

University of the Pacific
Arthur A. Dugoni School of Dentistry
2155 Webster Street
San Francisco, CA 94115
Phone: (415) 929-6425
dental.pacific.edu/

Colorado

University of Colorado at
Denver and Hlth Sci Ctr
School of Dentistry;
13065 E. 17th Avenue, F831P.O. Box 6508
Aurora, CO 80045
Phone: (303) 724-7100:
www.uchsc.edu/sod

Connecticut

University of Connecticut School of Dental Medicine
263 Farmington Avenue
Farmington, CT 06030
Phone: (860) 679- 2175
sdm.uchc.edu

Florida

Nova Southeastern University College of Dental Medicine

3200 S. University Drive

Fort Lauderdale, FL 33328

Phone: (954) 262-7311

dental.nova.edu

University of Florida College of Dentistry

1600 SW Archer Rd.

Rm D4-6

Gainesville, FL 32610

Phone: (352) 273-5800

www.dental.ufl.edu

Illinois

University of Illinois at Chicago College of Dentistry

801 South Paulina Street

Suite # 102

Chicago, IL 60612

Phone: (312) 996-1040

dentistry.uic.edu

Indiana

Indiana University School of Dentistry

1121 West Michigan Street

Indianapolis, IN 46202

Phone: (317) 274-7461

www.iusd.iupui.edu

Massachusetts

Boston University
Goldman School of Dental Medicine
Advanced Standing Program Admissions
Office of Admissions and Student Services
100 East Newton Street, Suite G 305
Boston, MA 02118
Phone: (617) 638-4787
dentalschool.bu.edu/admissions

Tufts University School of Dental Medicine
One Kneeland Street
Boston, MA 02111
Phone: (617) 636-6636
www.tufts.edu/dental

Maryland

University of Maryland Baltimore College of Dental Surgery
Office of Admissions
650 W. Baltimore Street
Room 6410 South
Baltimore, MD 21201
Phone: (410) 706-7472
www.dental.umaryland.edu

Michigan

University of Michigan School of Dentistry
1011 N. University Ave.
Ann Arbor, MI 48109
Phone: (734) 763-3311
www.dent.umich.edu

University of Detroit Mercy School of Dentistry
8200 W. Outer Dr.
MB 98
Detroit, MI 48219-3580
Phone: (313) 494-6621/20
www.udmercy.edu/dental

Minnesota

University of Minnesota
School of Dentistry
515 Delaware Street S.E.
15-131 Moos Tower
Minneapolis, MN 55455
Phone: (612)-625-6950
www.dentistry.umn.edu/programs_admissions/UMN_PASS.html

Missouri

University of Missouri-Kansas City School of Dentistry
650 East 25th Street
Kansas City, MO 64108

Phone: (816) 235-2010

www.umkc.edu/dentistry

Nebraska

University of Nebraska Medical Center College of Dentistry
40th & Holdrege Streets
Lincoln, NE 68583-0740
Phone: (402) 472-1301
www.unmc.edu/dentistry

Creighton University School of Dentistry
2500 California Plaza
Omaha, NE 68178-0240
Phone: (402) 280-5060
cudental.creighton.edu
(limited space available)

New Jersey

University of Medicine and Dentistry of New Jersey—New Jersey Dental School
Office of Admissions, Room B830
110 Bergen Street, PO Box 1709
Newark, NJ 07101-1709
Phone: 973-972-5362
dentalschool.umdnj.edu/

New York

State University of New York at Buffalo School of Dental Medicine

325 Squire Hall;

3435 Main Street

Buffalo, NY 14214-3008

Phone: (716) 829-2836

www.sdm.buffalo.edu

Columbia University College of Dental Medicine

630 West 168th Street – P&S Box 20

New York, NY 10032

Phone: (212) 305-3478

cpmcnet.columbia.edu/dept/dental

New York University College of Dentistry

345 East 24th Street

New York, NY 10010

Phone: (212) 998-9818

www.nyu.edu/dental/

State University of New York at Stony Brook School of Dental Medicine

Health Sciences Center

154 Rockland Hall

Stony Brook, NY 11794

Phone: (631) 632-8950

www.hsc.stonybrook.edu/dental

Ohio

Case Western Reserve Univ. School of Dental Medicine
10900 Euclid Avenue
Cleveland, OH 44106
Phone: (216) 368-3266
www.case.edu/dental/site/main.html

Pennsylvania

Temple University
The Maurice H. Kornberg School of Dentistry
3223 North Broad Street
Philadelphia, PA 19140
Phone: (215) 707-2799
www.temple.edu/dentistry

University of Pennsylvania
School of Dental Medicine
Robert Schattner Center
240 South 40th Street
Philadelphia, PA 19104-6030
Phone: (215) 898-0558
sdm-pass@pobox.upenn.edu
www.dental.upenn.edu

University of Pittsburgh
School of Dental Medicine
3501 Terrace Street
Pittsburgh, PA 15261

Phone: (412) 648-1938
www.dental.pitt.edu

Puerto Rico

University of Puerto Rico
School of Dentistry
Medical Sciences Campus
Main Building-Office #A103B, 1st Floor
San Juan, PR 00936-5067
Phone: (787) 758-2525, X1105
dental.rcm.upr.edu

Tennessee

University of Tennessee
College of Dentistry
University of Tennessee Health Science Ctr
875 Union Avenue
Memphis, TN 38163
Phone: (901) 448-6202
www.utmem.edu/dentistry

Texas

Univ. of Texas Hlth Sci Ctr-
Houston Dental Branch
6516 M. D. Anderson Blvd.,
Suite 155
Houston, TX 77030- 3402

Phone: (713) 500-4429

www.db.uth.tmc.edu

University of Texas Hlth Sci Ctr-
San Antonio Dental School
7703 Floyd Curl Drive
San Antonio, TX 78284
Phone: (210) 567-3160
www.dental.uthscsa.edu

Virginia

Virginia Commonwealth University School of Dentistry
P.O. Box 980566
520 North 12th Street
Richmond, VA 23298-0566
Phone: (804) 828-9184
www.dentistry.vcu.edu

Wisconsin

Marquette University School of Dentistry
1801 W. Wisconsin Avenue
Milwaukee, WI 53233
Phone: (414) 288-7485
www.dental.mu.edu

West Virginia

West Virginia University
School of Dentistry
Robert C. Byrd Hlth Sci Ctr.
1150 HSC North/Medical Center Drive;
Morgantown, WV 26506-9400
Phone: (304) 293-2521
www.hsc.wvu.edu/sod

DENTAL ETHICS

As the demand and popularity of dentists and dental procedures increases, there also is a great increase in the responsibility of dentists. Dentistry is a well-respected profession. And as we've discussed, there are a lot of great things about this profession. One of the greatest things is that a dentist can be his or her own boss. This autonomy is a great asset, which allows the dentist to control his or her work schedule, hiring, pay scale, and anything else that pertains to the practice. However, like in all health professions, especially in the United States, there is a huge need to make certain that the health profession applies professional principals and practical applications while being ethically and morally correct. This chapter focuses on the importance of ethics for a dentist as a health professional.

We all know that society is governed by rules and regulations. To be a dentist, you need to go to dental school, pass the National Boards, and then pass a licensing examination. Why all these exams? What is the purpose? These tests are in place to make sure that not only are you a competent dentist, but also that you will follow the rules and regulations of the profession. Each state may have different rules and it is important for every dentist to follow them.

Upon matriculation or prior to graduation, most health professionals take the Hippocratic Oath. Hippocrates was a Greek physician in 460 B.C. He is most well known for being the father of medicine. His prestige led him to be regarded the forefront physician of his time. He was one of the first ones to believe that bodily illness had a physical and rational explanation, and rejected that illness was caused by evil spirits or discontentment of the gods. However, his ethical beliefs led him to further illustrate the importance of treating the body as a whole, and not just as a body part (in our case, just a mouth). Prior to his death he founded a medical school and compiled an Oath of Medical Ethics, which today is known as the Hippocratic Oath.

The following is the modern version of the oath:[1]

I swear to fulfill, to the best of my ability and judgment, this covenant:

I will respect the hard-won scientific gains of those physicians in whose steps I walk, and gladly share such knowledge as is mine with those who are to follow.

I will apply, for the benefit of the sick, all measures which are required, avoiding those twin traps of overtreatment and therapeutic nihilism.

I will remember that there is art to medicine as well as science, and that warmth, sympathy, and understanding may outweigh the surgeon's knife or the chemist's drug.

I will not be ashamed to say "I know not," nor will I fail to call in my colleagues when the skills of another are needed for a patient's recovery.

I will respect the privacy of my patients, for their problems are not disclosed to me that the world may know. Most especially, must I tread with care in matters of life and death. If it is given me to save a life, all thanks. But it may also be within my power to take a life; this awesome responsibility must be faced with great humbleness and awareness of my own frailty. Above all, I must not play at God.

I will remember that I do not treat a fever chart, a cancerous growth, but a sick human being, whose illness may affect the person's family

---

[1] Written in 1964 by Louis Lasagna, Academic Dean of the School of Medicine at Tufts University, and used in many medical schools today.

and economic stability. My responsibility includes these related problems, if I am to care adequately for the sick.

ℬℭ

I will prevent disease whenever I can, for prevention is preferable to cure.

ℬℭ

I will remember that I remain a member of society, with special obligations to all my fellow human beings, those sound of mind and body as well as the infirm.

ℬℭ

If I do not violate this oath, may I enjoy life and art, respected while I live and remembered with affection thereafter. May I always act so as to preserve the finest traditions of my calling and may I long experience the joy of healing those who seek my help.

ℬ ℭ

Ethics for a pre-dental student:

In all professions there is a *code* one must follow. There are certain things you can do, and certain things you cannot do. When you knowingly do something that you are not supposed to do, that is supposed to be *unethical*. There are many ethical issues and dilemmas in the dental practice. In the beginning, you may ask yourself how this could be and in this portion, the goal is to acquaint the pre-dental student with an easily understood method for dental ethics. Also, during interviews many dental schools may ask you a question pertaining to dental ethics. It is your responsibility to understand and critically think about these questions when asked about them.

Professional obligation:

As a dentist, you have an obligation to provide excellent care for your patients and do anything that will increase their well-being. This means making hard decisions at times, putting patients first and profits and yourself second. Since dentists consider themselves *professionals,* they must act in a professional manner. A professional is anyone who possesses a unique understanding and expertise in a specific area and puts their skills into practice. The American Dental Association's Code of Ethics says, "Qualities of compassion, kindness, integrity, fairness and charity complement the ethical practice of dentistry and help to define the true professional."

Terms you should know:

Many people consider that the terms *moral* and *ethical* mean two different things. Moral is defined as teaching or exhibiting goodness or correctness of character and behavior, and ethics is defined as: A theory or a system of moral values. So, we can illustrate both these terms to be synonyms or the same thing.

Code of Ethics in a Nutshell:

- ➢ The dentist should respect the patient's confidentiality.
- ➢ The dentist should do everything not to harm the patient, or keep the patient from harming him/herself.
- ➢ The dentist should do everything in his/her ability for the patient's social welfare.
- ➢ The dentist should treat people fairly.
- ➢ The dentist should be truthful.

What you should know about patient confidentiality:

In all health professions, patient confidentiality is regarded as one of the most important obligations. Dentists, as well as all other health professionals, know many aspects of patients' lives and behavior. This can include: sexual orientation, drug habits, diseases (including HIV, STD's, etc.), medication history, and family history (including abuse, diseases in family, etc.). For this reason, it is very important that a dentist respect the patient and his or her lifestyle. There is definitely a sense of trust that develops between a health professional and the patient, due to the fact a patient knows that a health professional is obliged to keep what is discussed between them confidential.

It is the duty of the dentist to preserve a patient's privacy at all circumstances. Protecting privacy is a vital skill that any health professional must learn to handle. It is important to respect those that you serve and understand the role you play in the patient's life. Patients will tell you things that even their best friends or spouses don't know. For this reason, it is important not to disclose any information outside the vicinity of the original conversation.

Privacy for HIV/AIDS patients:

The terms HIV and AIDS are not easy words to hear, especially in a setting which involves exposure to blood and bodily fluids. One reason there is an increased awareness of privacy for individuals with HIV or other immune suppressed diseases is the social implications and stereotypes associated with these diseases. However, if a professional knows about the HIV/AIDS status of a patient, then it is a must to keep that information confidential if the patient deems it private. Health professionals, in general, including dentists, need to know of a patient's HIV status to properly treat them. If a patient knew that there might be a breach of privacy, the less lenient they would be to share that information.

Avoiding harm to patient:

As with all health professionals, the goal is to protect the patient and his/her welfare. For this reason, it is imperative for a dental health professional to do everything in his or her power to prevent any harm from coming to the patient. That means sterilizing the instruments, changing syringe heads, wearing clean gloves, and keeping the room sanitary to avoid cross contamination. If there is a discrepancy, it should be the dentist's responsibility to inform the patient immediately. For example, if by chance a used needle was used on a patient and the dentist has knowledge of this error, the dentist must inform the patient of the error and take appropriate measures to ensure that the patient was not harmed (do a HIV-serotype test, Hepatitis B tests, etc).

Protecting the Patient:

As a health professional, dentistry requires the dentist to be involved with all aspects of a patient's life. During a check up, the dentist may ask questions which one would think that are not pertaining to dentistry. But remember that Hippocrates thought about treating a person as a whole, not just a body part. For this reason, the dentist may ask questions like:

- Family history of disease (deaths, diseases)
- History of medications
- Drug allergies
- Allergies
- Other medical problems
- Eating habits
- Sleeping Habits
- Brushing habits
- Recent sickness
- Other social activities/stresses (weddings, jobs, children, buying a house, etc.)

Usually, a dentist compiles a mental picture and is more aware of the patient's lifestyle, history, and certain implications. For example, the patient may tell the dentist about hypertension in the family and a dentist may observe symptoms of hypertension in the oral cavity, and then guide the patient with that information.

Treating patients fairly:

It is a simple rule that if you treat people well, they will come back to you. This is nothing but the truth in a dental atmosphere. A dentist must treat a patient humanely and compassionately. There should be a definite bonding between patient and dentist and this dentist-patient relationship should always be kept in high regards. If a patient lacks trust in the dentist, then there is a question as to why a certain procedure is being done. This lack of confidence can bring a lot of trouble and unneeded tension, ending up into disputes and even legal problems. So it is imperative that a dentist treat everyone equally in all aspects.

Honesty, the best policy:

"Oh, what a tangled web we weave, when first we practice to deceive." Sir Walter Scott says it eloquently enough to illustrate that deception is unacceptable for any health professional. Deception is misleading the patient, the staff, the insurance company, or anything else that demeans the dental profession. It is up to each individual dentist to keep high standards of professional conduct. There are always hard circumstances that one must learn to face. As a health professional, you must remember your main purpose: to help the patient. This may mean telling the patient something they do not want to hear. Honesty is always best. Lying will only complicate your life and disgrace the profession. The complexities of dental ethics are never ending. However, if you understand the simple rules above you should be able to tackle most interview questions regarding dental ethics. Also, understanding the above rules will help you during observation or shadowing in a dental office. Each state has its own regulations and you should also check those out as well. It would not be a bad idea if you could sit down with the dentist you are working with and ask them the rules of your state and if they could share any insights on ethics, etc.

If you have read this chapter and understand ethical issues, we have compiled some situations to think about. Ask yourself these questions and see how you could approach them differently.

Questions in Dental Ethics:
1) You have a friend who just moved into your town and is looking for a dentist. You recommend him to your dentist and he went in for a cleaning. During the examination, your dentist noticed that many of his previous dental procedures were done inaccurately or unnecessarily. What do you think the professional obligation of your dentist is?

    • Should he ignore it and just move on?

    • Should he ask questions regarding the procedures?

2) If your uncle went to your dentist and your dentist noticed a *lump* growing in the posterior mouth, is it the dentist's responsibility to tell your uncle? The lump may be cancer; however a dentist does not treat cancer.

3) If you are volunteering for a dentist and she wanted you to extract the molar, should you do it?

4) If a patient comes into the office interested in bleaching their teeth, and if their insurance does not cover bleaching since it fits into "cosmetics," should the dentist go ahead and give the patient what she asks and charge the insurance under a different procedure?

5) A non-English speaking patient comes into your clinic for an extraction. During the procedure, the dentist goes ahead and does a root canal therapy instead without telling the patient. Is this ethical?

6) If an HIV-positive patient comes in and the dentist knows about the suppressed immune status of the patient, should the dentist do anything differently in treatment?

7) If you know a patient is HIV-positive, should you sterilize the instruments more than once?

8) A dentist knows of a better therapy for a patient, but does not perform it, as he knows the patient's insurance will not cover it. Is suppressing the information and doing a less effective therapy ethical?

9) If a patient comes in smelling of tobacco smoke, does the dentist have a professional obligation to warn the patient of the dangers of such activity?

10) During an initial examination, should the dentist ask about the overall health of the patient, including medications they are taking, even if certain questions do not pertain exactly to dentistry?

11) In a situation with a young child who is uncooperative, should the dentist make-up "white lies" in order to calm the child and make him/her cooperative?

☼ ☙

BIBLIOGRAPHY

AMERICAN ASSOCIATION OF DENTAL SCHOOLS. 2000. *Admission Requirements of United States and Canadian Dental Schools: Entering Class of 2001,* 38th edition. Washington, DC: American Association of Dental Schools.

WEAVER, RICHARD G.; HADEN, N. KARL; and VALACHOVIC, RICHARD W. 2000. "U.S. Dental School Applicants and Enrollees: A Ten Year Perspective." *Journal of Dental Education* 64:867–874.

INTERNET RESOURCES

AMERICAN DENTAL ASSOCIATION. 2000. "Dental Admission Testing Program"
.... www.ada.org/prof/ed/testing/dat.asp

AMERICAN DENTAL ASSOCIATION. 2001. "National Board Dental Examination Program"
................................www.ada.org/prof/prac/licensure/lic-natbd.html

CANADIAN DENTAL ASSOCIATION, 2009. "Scope of Dental Admission Test"
.... www.cda-adc.ca/en/dental_profession/dat/information

ಐ ಞ

SOME USEFUL LINKS FOR PRE-DENTAL STUDENTS

American Dental Assoc (ADA) .... www.ada.org

American Dental Education Association (ADEA) ... www.adea.org

American Student Dental Association (ASDA) ...www.asdanet.org

Associated American Dental Schools Application Service
 (AADSAS)................................. https://portal.aadsasweb.org

Hispanic Dental Association (HDA) .... www.hdassoc.org

National Dental Association (NDA) \ .... www.ndaonline.org

National Institute of Dental and Craniofacial Research (NIDCR)
 .... www.nidcr.nih.gov

Student Doctor Network® .... www.studentdoctor.net

The Student Doctor Network® Pre-Dental Discussion Forum
 ..... http://forums.studentdoctor.net/forumdisplay.php?f=17

Dental Admissions Test Materials......................... www.datpat.com

INDEX

A

AADSAS · 41, 46, 93
about dental schools · 85
academic difficulty · 119
academic score · 91
acceptance checklist · 121
acceptance letter · 98
acceptance notification · 98
ADEA · 41, 46
Administered by American Dental Education Association · 46
admission essay, importance · 95
admission scores, DAT/GPA · 88
Advanced Education in General Dentistry · 110, 112
advanced standing program · 114
Advanced Standing Programs · 187
AEGD · 110, 112
AIDS patients · 202
American Dental Education Association · 93
angle ranking · 21
application cycle · 8
application fee · 96
application for DAT · 89
application process · 45
application timeline · 86
application, Canadian · 70
application, dental · 43
application, non-traditional · 61
application, online · 46
application, post-baccalaureate · 63
application, pre-requisites · 93
application, secondary · 96
application, submitting · 44
application, Texas schools · 46
application, tracking · 49
Associated American Dental Schools Application Service · 46

B

before dental school, after acceptance · 101
bibliography · 207
biology · 13, 71

C

Canadian applicants · 70
chemistry · 13, 72
choosing school · 115
clinically oriented school · 109
college · 9, 11
college major · 11, 85
college, required courses · 12, 13
competition · 93
completing your degree · 100
confidentiality · 201
core classes · 14
Cost of Attendance sheet · 178
cost of education · 118
courses, recommended · 101
cube counting · 23

D

D.D.S. · 102, 108

D.M.D. · 102, 108
DAT · 12, 14, 16, 86
DAT important sections · 90
DAT location · 92
DAT on computer · 35
DAT preparation · 32, 39
DAT retake · 42
DAT scheduling · 92
DAT scores · 41, 92
DAT sections · 90
DAT special accommodations · 92
DAT subjects · 25
DAT vs GPA vs PAT · 41
DAT, Canadian · 71
DAT, Canadian vs American · 89
DAT, mandatory · 89
DAT, retake · 91
DAT/GPA · 88
debt · 177
December 1st · 98
Dental Admission Test · 12
Dental Admissions Test · 14, 16
Dental Aptitude Test, Canadian · 71
dental essay · 50
dental school, first two years · 103
dental school, length of study · 103
dental school, third and fourth years · 104
dental schools · 95
dental schools, organization · 108
Dentariae Medicinae Doctor · 103
dentist, foreign-trained · 114
dexterity · 71, 101
dexterity, improving · 102
doctorate program · 110

E

early application · 95
empathy · 11

endodontics · 104
English class · 13
environment, study · 33
essay · 50
essay, admission · 95
essay, sample · 52, 55, 57, 59
ethical issues · 200
ethics · 83, 198
ethics questions · 204
exam, regional board · 112
exam, state board · 112
experience · 9, 87
experience, dental · 87

F

faculty, dental school · 118
FAFSA · 180
fairness · 203
FAQ · 85
FFELP · 179
FICO score · 178
financial aid · 178
financing · 177
foreign-trained dentist · 114, 186
further training · 110

G

general dentist · 105
general practice residency · 110
General Practice Residency · 112
glossary · 123
GPA · 14, 15, 40, 41, 70
GPR · 110, 112
grades do matter · 100
grades, importance · 88
grading in dental school · 108
grading, pass-fail · 109

H

hands, large · 102
Health Professions Student Loan · 179
high school · 9
Hippocratic Oath · 198
HIV patients · 202
hobbies · 11
hole punching · 22
honesty · 204
housing · 121
HPSL · 179

I

intensity of school · 117
International Dental Candidates · 186
internet resources · 207
internet resources, pre-dental · 208
interview · 8, 74, 97
interview attire · 98
interview length · 98
interview, length · 116

K

Kaplan · 12
keyholes · 19

L

learning disability, documented · 119
length of interview · 98
lists of programs · 65

loan
    consolidate · 180
    Health Professions Student · 179
    Perkins · 179
    private · 180
    Stafford · 179

M

male to female ration in dental schools · 93
math class · 13
Military Scholarship · 180
multiple school offers · 99

N

National Dental Board Exam · 110
National Health Service Corps · 180
National Loan Data System · 177
NDBE · 106, 107, 110
NERB · 112
NHSC · 180
non-traditional applicant · 61
Northeast Regional Board · 112

O

obligation
    professional · 200
optimal application · 95
oral and maxillofacial surgery · 104
oral maxillofacial surgery · 107
oral pathology · 105
oral radiology · 105
orthodontics · 104, 107
outside interests · 11

P

paper folding · 24
PAT importance · 91
PAT sample problems · 19
PAT score · 91
pedodontics · 104, 107
perceptual ability · 72
Perceptual Ability Test · 17
periodontics · 104
Perkins Loan · 179
personal essay · 50
personality · 88
physics · 13
post-baccalaureate programs · 63
post-doctorate programs · 106
pre-dental · 8, *9*
prerequisites for admission · 85
Princeton · 12
privacy, patient · 202
private loan · 180
program, advanced standing · 114
programs, general · 64, 66
programs, master's degree · 67
programs, post-baccalaureate · 67
prosthodontics · 105
protect the patient · 202

Q

quantitative analysis · 35
questions · 50
questions about dental schools · 85
questions, college · 79
questions, common interview · 75
questions, dental aptitude · 77
questions, ethics · 83
questions, program-related · 82
questions, sample interview · 76
questions, volunteer · 81
questions, work experience · 81

R

reading comprehension · 72
re-application · 115
recommendation letter · 43
recommended courses · 101
regional board exam · 112
relax · 101
requirements, college · 12
research experience · 87
research experience, importance · 107
research-oriented school · 109
residency · 104, 106, 107
residency, general practice · 110
review materials · 12

S

schedule, study · 34
scholarship
    military · 180
    National Health Service Corps · 180
school schedule · 14
school, choosing a · 115
schools
    Alabama · 139
    Arizona · 139
    California · 141
    Canada · 138
    Colorado · 145
    Connecticut · 146
    District of Columbia · 146
    Florida · 147
    Illinois · 148

Indiana · 150
Iowa · 150
Kentucky · 151
Maryland · 153
Massachusetts · 153
Michigan · 156
Minnesota · 157
Missouri · 158
Nebraska · 159
Nevada · 160
New Jersey · 161
New York · 161
North Carolina · 164
Ohio · 164
Oklahoma · 166
Oregon · 166
Pennsylvania · 167
Puerto Rico · 169
South Carolina · 170
Tennessee · 170
Texas · 171
United States · 136
Virginia · 173
Washington · 174
West Virginia · 175
Wisconsin · 175
scores, DAT · 90, 92
secondary application · 96
sections of DAT · 90
shadowing · 9, 87
specializing · 105
specialties, dental · 104
specialty training · 106
specialty, competitive · 107
Stafford Loan · 179
state board exam · 112

study environment · 33
study schedule · 34
study schedule, sample · 36
survey, natural sciences
    biology content · 26
    general chemistry · 27
    organic chemistry · 31

T

terminology · 123
testing in dental school · 119
Thompson Prometric · 92
Thomson Prometeric · 89
time period, application · 94
timeline · 86
TOEFL · 114
training, specialty · 106
travel expenses · 97

V

volunteer · 11, 81

W

working while in dental school · 120

Y

your top choice · 99

NOTES

Notes

Notes

NOTES

Notes

Notes

Notes

Notes

Notes

Notes

NOTES

Notes

www.ingramcontent.com/pod-product-compliance
Lightning Source LLC
Chambersburg PA
CBHW020652230426
43665CB00008B/411